Adult-Gerontology and Family Nurse Practitioner

Adult-Gerontology and Family Nurse Practitioner

Craig Sorkin, APN
Riverside Medical Group
Jersey City, New Jersey

Elizabeth August, MD
CMO Bergen County
Riverside Medical Group
Hackensack, New Jersey

Conrad Fischer, MD
Residency Program Director
Brookdale University Medical Center
New York, New York
Associate Professor of Medicine, Physiology and
  Pharmacology, Touro College of Medicine

McGraw Hill Education

New York   Chicago   San Francisco   Athens   London   Madrid
Mexico City   Milan   New Delhi   Singapore   Sydney   Toronto

1 2 3 4 5 6 7 8 9   ROV   21 20 19 18 17 16

ISBN 978-0-07-183439-1
MHID 0-07-183439-7

This book was set in Minion pro by Cenveo® Publisher Services.
The editors were Susan Barnes and Christina M. Thomas.
The production supervisor was Richard Ruzycka.
Project management was provided by Kritika Kaushik, Cenveo Publisher Services.
The cover designer was Dreamit, Inc.
RR Donnelley was printer and binder.

This book is printed on acid-free paper.

Library of Congress Cataloging-in-Publication Data

Names: Sorkin, Craig, author. | August, Elizabeth V., author. | Fischer, Conrad, author.
Title: Adult-gerontology and family nurse practitioner / Craig Sorkin, Elizabeth August, Conrad Fischer.
Description: New York : McGraw-Hill Education, [2017] | Includes index.
Identifiers: LCCN 2016003886| ISBN 9780071834391 (pbk. : alk. paper) |
    ISBN 0071834397 (pbk. : alk. paper)
Subjects: MESH: Nursing Care | Advanced Practice Nursing | Nurse Practitioners |
Test Taking Skills | Problems and Exercises
Classification: LCC RT42 | NLM WY 18.2 | DDC 610.73—dc23 LC record available at http://lccn.loc.gov/2016003886

McGraw-Hill books are available at special quantity discounts to use as premiums and sales promotions, or for use in corporate training programs. To contact a representative, please visit the Contact Us pages at www.mhprofessional.com.

This book is dedicated to my family, friends, mentors, and everyone who has supported me throughout this project and every other I have undertaken.

A special thank-you to my wonderful Wife, Jessica Taubman-Sorkin, and my coauthors, Elizabeth August and Conrad Fischer, without all of whom I could not have completed this book.

Contents

Preface

This book will serve to prepare and polish your knowledge in preparation for your board exam. This book has material that will serve for both Adult-Gerontology and Family Nurse Practitioner exams to be used as needed. It is advised that you take the material at face value and make notes to yourself to enhance further studying. Use this book as a study guide and outline to brush up on topics that are most commonly assessed on the board exams. The case questions, exam tips, and clinical tips throughout each chapter provide simple, concise information that is most relevant to clinical practice and to passing the exam. The tests at the end of the book serve as practice exams and provide suggestions as to where more practice, reading, and knowledge growth are required.

ENJOY! And good studying.

Introduction to the AANP and ANCC Examinations

Congratulations on nearing completion of your adult or family nurse practitioner program! This is the beginning of a very exciting and rewarding career.

THE AMERICAN ACADEMY OF NURSE PRACTITIONERS EXAM

The American Academy of Nurse Practitioners (AANP) certifies graduates of accredited Master of Science in Nursing (MSN) programs in three categories: Adult, Geriatric, and Family Nurse Practitioner. Note that the adult and geriatric categories have now been combined into the designation of adult-gerontology primary care nurse practitioner. The AANP is an independent certification organization accredited through the National Commission for Certifying Agencies (NCCA).

The AANP exam consists of 150 questions, 15 of which are experimental practice questions that do not count toward your final grade. You have 3 hours to complete the exam.

The passing score for the exam is 66%. As of 2015, the passing rate for each section is as follows: Adult Nurse Practitioner 80%, Family Nurse Practitioner 87.3%, and Geriatric Nurse Practitioner 88.9%.

Question Breakdown

The AANP exam follows the nurse practitioner model in that its question cover the categories of assessment, diagnosis, plan, and evaluation. The knowledge base required is as follows:

1. Health promotion and disease prevention
2. Anatomy, physiology, and pathophysiology
3. Interviewing concepts and techniques
4. Health history
5. Signs and symptoms
6. Physical examination
7. Laboratory/diagnostic tests
8. Clinical decision making
9. Differential diagnosis
10. Pharmacological therapies
11. Nonpharmacological/complementary/alternative therapies
12. Diagnostic and therapeutic procedures

13. Biopsychosocial theories
14. Patient and family education and counseling
15. Community resources
16. Healthcare economics and practice management
17. Evidence-based practice
18. Legal and ethical issues
19. Cultural competence
20. Principles of epidemiology

THE AMERICAN NURSES CREDENTIALING CENTER EXAM

The American Nurses Credentialing Center (ANCC) is affiliated with the American Nurses Association. It offers Adult, Geriatric, and Family Nurse Practitioner exams as well as many others. The ANCC exam consists of 175 questions, 25 of which are practice questions that do not count toward your final grade. You have 3 hours to complete the exam. The ANCC exam includes clinical, research, and legal questions.

A big difference between the AANP and ANCC exams is that the AANP exam gives lab test ranges, whereas the ANCC exam does not. The AANP exam is also more clinically focused than the ANCC exam.

The passing score for the ANCC exam is 350 points out of a possible 500. The passing rate for each section is as follows: Adult Nurse Practitioner 81%, Geriatric Nurse Practitioner 85.5%, and Family Nurse Practitioner 80.5%.

Question Breakdown

The ANCC exam question breakdown is as follows:

- Clinical management: 34%
- Professional roles and policy: 6%
- The nurse practitioner and patient relationship: 11%
- The assessment of acute and chronic illnesses: 26%
- Research: 2%
- Health promotion and disease prevention: 21%

THE EXAM PROCESS

Both the AANP and ANCC exams are recognized throughout the United States. There is no definitive answer as to whether one is better or whether one is more highly regarded by employers. Both exams are computer based and scored electronically. Both credentialing organizations allow students to retake the exam should they not pass on the first attempt. Both organizations will forward your scores to your state boards for you if you sign a release form allowing them to do so.

It is important to stay on top of the paperwork involved in obtaining your advanced practice nurse license. The process is cumbersome but manageable if you are aware of all the guidelines required for licensure.

Remember that every state has different requirements. Most of the information you will need will be available on the website of your state's board of nursing. Make sure to pay attention to all the requirements of your state's board, not just the schooling requirements.

1

Health Promotion and Disease Prevention

PREVENTION IS CATCHING PATHOLOGY BEFORE IT HAPPENS

- Creating a healthy lifestyle to prevent disease
  - Educating our patients on diet and exercise to prevent obesity
  - Smoking cessation education to prevent lung cancer

Secondary Prevention Is Catching Pathology Early

- Mammograms to catch breast cancer early
- Pap smears to catch cervical cancer early
- Colonoscopies to catch colon cancer early

Tertiary Prevention Is the Rehabilitation (Rehab) Phase

- The event happened; now, how do we prevent it from worsening or reoccurring?
  - Effective glucose control in patients with diabetes to prevent worsening neuropathy or nephropathy

Screening Exams

- Annual physical examination.
- Obstetrics and gynecology (OB/GYN) exam and Pap smear every 1-3 years starting at age 21, regardless of sexual activity. Perform every 5 years if combined with HPV testing. Screening stops at age 65.
- Mammogram every 1-2 years starting at age 50 or 10 years earlier than the youngest family member with breast cancer.
- Colonoscopy every 10 years starting at age 50 or 10 years earlier than the youngest family member with colon cancer or age 40, whichever is earlier.

Antibiotic Usage

- Once you pass your board exams and are licensed, the decision to prescribe is up to you.
- Remember that antibiotic resistance is a growing problem.

■ Remember the signs and symptoms of bacterial versus viral infections (such as fever, type of discharge, and speed of presenting symptoms), and prescribe accordingly.

The United States Preventive Services Task Force has an excellent website consisting of the most up-to-date recommendations for pathology screening. You will likely not see this material on an exam, but it is valuable for your future practice. See www.uspreventiveservicestaskforce.org.

2
Pediatrics

A. RASHES

AA. Kawasaki Disease

- Kawasaki disease is an inflammatory disorder of the blood vessels.
- The disease usually occurs in children under the age of 5.
- It can affect the blood vessels, skin, mucous membranes, lymph nodes, and, in severe cases, the heart and coronary vessels.

Presentation

- High and persistent fever (tends not to respond to antipyretics) that lasts 5 or more days
- Irritability
- Red tongue ("strawberry tongue")
- Edematous, cracking lips
- Lymphadenopathy (Figure 2-1)
- Erythema of the palms of the hands and soles of the feet
- Maculopapular body rash
- Diarrhea
- Myocarditis and/or pericarditis

Diagnosis

There is no specific laboratory test for Kawasaki disease. Diagnosis is based upon clinical history, which must include the following:

- Fever for 5 or more days plus 4 of the 5 following criteria:
  - Erythema of the lips or mouth
  - Body rash
  - Swelling or redness of the hands and feet
  - Red eyes
  - Lymphadenopathy

Diagnostic testing is not used for diagnosis; however, an elevation in the white blood cells (WBC) and an elevation in inflammatory panels (erythrocyte sedimentation rate [ESR] and C-reactive protein [CRP]) are seen in the bloodwork.

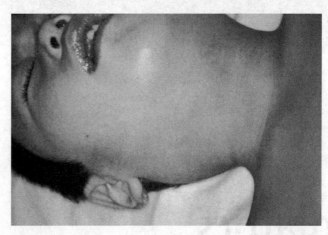

FIGURE 2-1 Kawasaki disease. Note the cervical lymphadenopathy. Reproduced with permission from Knoop K, Stack L, Storrow A, et al: *The Atlas of Emergency Medicine*, 3rd ed. New York, NY: McGraw-Hill, Inc; 2010. Photo contributor: Tomisaku Kawasaki, MD.

Treatment

Children with Kawasaki disease should be hospitalized. Pediatric cardiology, rheumatology, and infectious disease specialists should be consulted to assist with care. Cardiologist should be consulted as the disease can affect the heart; rheumatologist should be consulted as the disease can affect the muscles, ligaments, and joint structures; and, for infectious disease specialist should be consulted to guide antimicrobial therapy.

A transthoracic echocardiogram should be done to assess for coronary artery aneurysms. Intravenous immunoglobulin (IVIG) and aspirin are the standard of care for the treatment of Kawasaki disease. Aspirin helps to prevent coronary artery aneurysms.

Complications

The most feared complication with Kawasaki disease is coronary artery aneurysms. These are most likely to occur in patients with the following characteristics:

- Under the age of 1 year or over the age of 9 years
- Male sex
- A fever lasting more than 14 days
- Hyponatremia
- An elevated WBC count
- A low hematocrit

In order to monitor for these complications, an echocardiogram should be done, and a referral to pediatric cardiology should be made.

AB. Coxsackievirus

Coxsackievirus, types A and B, is a viral syndrome of the *Picornaviridae* family. This syndrome, also called "hand, foot, and mouth disease," is caused by a virus that produces painful blisters in the oropharynx and on the palms of the hands and soles of the feet. Lesions are usually described as itchy or painful vesicles (Figure 2-2).

Diagnosis

Diagnosis of Coxsackievirus is based on the clinical presentation of fever with rash. Immunoglobulin G (IgG) and immunoglobulin M (IgM) panels can be completed for Coxsackie A and B but are not needed if a clinical diagnosis can be made.

Referral

Severe cases can produce hemorrhagic conjunctivitis (inflammation and erythema of the conjunctiva), aseptic meningitis, and paralysis.

EXAM TIP
Strawberry tongue and high fever are hallmarks of Kawasaki disease.

CLINICAL TIP
- Fever precedes blisters.
- Blisters are itchy and appear on the hands, feet, and mouth.

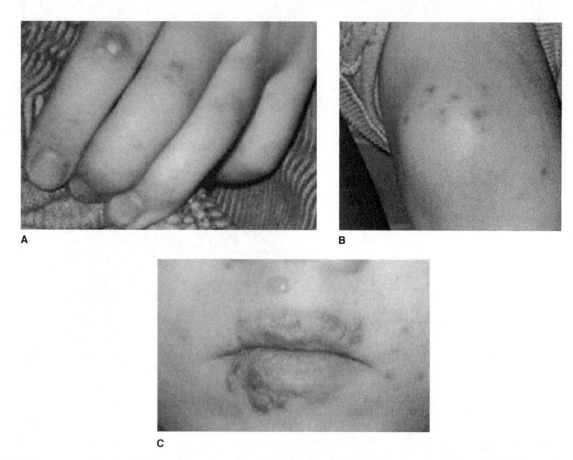

A

B

C

FIGURE 2-2 Fever precedes the blisters and can last for 7-10 days. Used with permission from Centers for Disease Control and Prevention/Emerging Infectious Diseases.

AC. Measles

Measles is a viral syndrome caused by *Morbillivirus*, a member of the Paramyxoviri-dae family. Measles is characterized by fever, cough, rhinitis, and then a rash with small white spots in the mouth (referred to as Koplik spots or Koplik's sign).

There are 5 stages of infection:

1. The **incubation period** lasts 6-19 days and is the most contagious stage. Patients are contagious for 5 days *before* the rash appears through 4 days *after* the rash appears.

2. The **prodrome** is the stage when symptoms begin to appear, including
   a. Fever
   b. Malaise
   c. Anorexia
   d. Conjunctivitis
   e. Coryza (congestion, postnasal drip, and rhinitis)
   f. Cough

3. **Enanthem** is the appearance of Koplik spots (white, gray, or blueish spots 1-3 mm in diameter on a red base seen in the mouth), which disappear as the rash develops. Koplik spots are pathognomonic of measles, meaning that they are indicative of measles (Figure 2-3).

4. **Exanthem** is a maculopapular rash that begins on the face and spreads down-ward. It starts in the center of the body and spreads outward (Figure 2-4). The rash will blanch in the beginning but will stop toward the end. Petechiae may be present. The rash usually spares the palms of the hands and the soles of the feet.

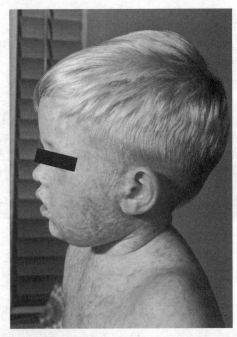

FIGURE 2-3 Measles Koplik's spots. Used with permission from Public Health Image Library, Centers for Disease Control and Prevention.

EXAM TIP

Measles is an airborne virus that spreads via cough, sneezing, saliva, and nasal secretions.

CLINICAL TIP

If Koplik spots are seen, the patient has measles.

CLINICAL TIP

Severe cases of measles can produce diarrhea, blindness, meningitis, encephalitis (an inflammation of the brain), and pneumonia.

The other symptoms of measles peak during the rash stage. The fever will peak 2-3 days after the appearance of the rash. Clinical improvement usually occurs 48 hours after the rash.

5. **Recovery** occurs following the exathem stage. A cough may persist for the following 1-2 weeks.

Vaccination for measles is included in the measles, mumps, and rubella (MMR) vaccine, which is given at ages 1 and 6 years. Vaccination has decreased the incidence of measles by 75%, although the recent rise in non-vaccination has caused a resurgence of this infection.

Diagnosis

The diagnosis of measles is clinical. IgG/IgM panels can be completed to confirm diagnosis. The patient will likely have a clinical history of fever for 3-4 days, cough, coryza, and conjunctivitis.

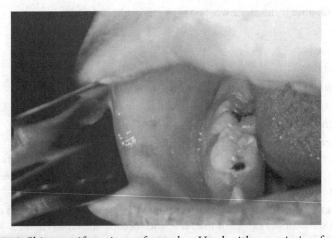

FIGURE 2-4 Skin manifestations of measles. Used with permission from the Centers for Disease Control and Prevention.

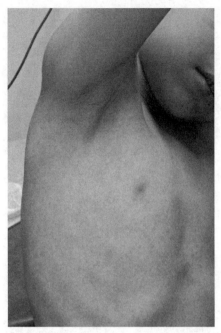

FIGURE 2-5 Skin manifestations scarlett fever. Reproduced with permission from Richard P. Usatine, MD and Usatine RP, Smith MA, Chumley HS, et al. *The Color Atlas of Family Medicine*, 2nd ed. New York, NY: McGraw-Hill; 2013.

Treatment

Treatment for measles is supportive:

- Control temperature with acetaminophen and ibuprofen
- Hydration

Antibiotics are indicated only for confirmed or suspected cases of bacterial infection (eg, pneumonia, conjunctivitis, meningitis).

AD. Scarlet Fever

Scarlet fever is a bacterial infection caused by group A *Streptococcus*. It is a mild illness that can be easily treated with antibiotics. It usually affects children aged 5-12 years. Group A *Streptococcus* spreads via droplets and is contagious to others. If scarlet fever is not treated, it may lead to long-term complications, such as rheumatic fever or renal complications.

Physical Exam

The rash that appears with scarlet fever is very typical: it appears first on the neck and face, then spreads to the chest and back (Figure 2-5). Hyperpigmentation can occur in patients with a darker skin tone. The rash has a sandpaper texture. Table 2-1 lists the signs and symptoms of scarlet fever.

CLINICAL TIP
- Fever precedes rash
- Flat rash starting on face
- Fever for 3-4 days

EXAM TIP
Know what Koplik spots are.

TABLE 2-1	Signs and Symptoms of Scarlet Fever
Fever	
Sore throat	
Red tongue with strawberry appearance (Figure 2-6)	
Red spots on soft palate (Forchheimer spots)	
Rash: blanches with pressure, sandpaper texture, worse in folds	
Skin peeling after rash starts to fade	

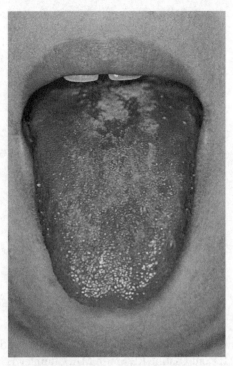

FIGURE 2-6 Strawberry tongue. Reproduced with permission from Wolff K, Johnson R, Saavedra AP. *Fitzpatrick's Color Atlas and Synopsis of Clinical Dermatology*, 7th ed. New York, NY: McGraw-Hill; 2013.

Diagnosis

The clinical diagnosis of scarlet fever is made based on signs and symptoms. However, some diagnostic tests may be positive if completed:

- Elevated WBC count
- Elevated inflammatory panels (ESR and CRP)
- Antistreptolysin O titer elevation

Treatment

Penicillin and macrolide antibiotics are the first line of treatment for scarlet fever. Recent resistance has been noted with some antibiotics, such as erythromycin.

Prevention

There is no vaccination for group A *Streptococcus*; however, there are ways to prevent an infection. Handwashing is the best option and should be done often. Also avoid sharing utensils, linens, towels, and toothbrushes. Children diagnosed with strep throat or scarlet fever should stay home for 24 hours after beginning antibiotics.

AE. Fifth Disease

Erythema infectiosum, otherwise known as fifth disease or "slapped-cheek fever," is a virus caused by parvovirus B19. Parvovirus B19 belongs to the *Erythroparvovirus* genus within the Parvoviridae family.

Presentation

- Usually school-aged children
- Fever
- Headache
- Rash

EXAM TIP

Look for a question discussing a child who has the following signs:
- Sandpaper-like rash
- Fever

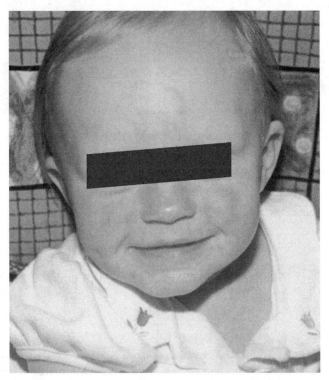

FIGURE 2-7 Slapped cheek appearance of Parvovirus. Reproduced with permission from Kasper D, Fauci A, Hauser S. *Harrison's Principles of Internal Medicine*, 19th ed. New York, NY: McGraw-Hill; 2015.

- Cold-like signs and symptoms (ie, runny nose, cough, congestion)
- Rash is bright red on the cheeks and occasionally spreads down the face to the torso and arms

The nonspecific symptoms of fifth disease are indicated in the prodromal stage and at the onset of viremia. Two to five days later, the rash will appear on the face (Figure 2-7). The lace-like rash that appears on the torso and extremities occurs several days after the facial rash appears.

Diagnosis

- A diagnosis is made from the clinical history and physical.
- Patients will present with a fever and typical rash.
- IgG/IgM panels can be completed for a conclusive diagnosis; these are mostly done in pregnant patients when it is imperative to know if they have immunity.

Treatment

- Treatment is supportive: acetaminophen and ibuprofen for pain and fever control.

CLINICAL TIP
There are 5 syndromes associated with parvovirus B19:
- Erythema infectiosum (most likely tested)
- Arthropathy
- Transient aplastic crisis
- Fetal infection (during pregnancy)
- Red blood cell aplasia in immunocompromised patients

CLINICAL AND EXAM TIP
- "Slapped-face" rash on the cheeks

B. CONGENITAL MALFORMATIONS

BA. Tetralogy of Fallot

Tetralogy of Fallot is a congenital anatomic cardiac abnormality. There are 4 (hence "tetralogy") different abnormalities:

- Pulmonary artery stenosis
- Large overriding aorta (meaning it is partially on the right side)
- Ventricular septal defect
- Right ventricular hypertrophy

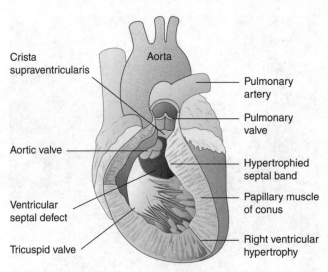

FIGURE 2-8 Tetralogy of Fallot. Reproduced with permission from Doherty GM. *CURRENT Diagnosis & Treatment: Surgery*, 14th ed. New York, NY: McGraw-Hill; 2015.

Tetralogy of Fallot is the most common *cyanotic* heart defect to occur during the first year of life and occurs equally in both genders. It a sporadic defect. As a result of right-to-left shunting (abnormal blood flow) through the ventricular septal defect, there is a decrease in the amount of oxygenated blood circulating in the body (Figure 2-8).

Presentation

Children with tetralogy of Fallot will present with cyanosis and failure to thrive. The symptoms can appear any time from the newborn period until childhood, depending on the severity of the defect. Affected children will often experience "tet spells." Tet spells may occur in the newborn stage when the infant becomes agitated or in childhood when the child is running or playing. A tet spell is characterized by a sudden onset of cyanosis, noted particularly in the fingertips or around the lips. If the child is old enough to be walking or running, he or she will often squat down, which helps increase blood flow back to the heart.

Physical Exam

Tetralogy of Fallot is characterized by a crescendo–decrescendo, harsh systolic murmur, best heard along the left sternal border.

Diagnosis

An echocardiogram is the most accurate test for Tetralogy of Fallot. If a chest X-ray is done, a boot-shaped heart will be seen.

Treatment

Surgical repair of the abnormal structures is the only treatment for Tetralogy of Fallot.

BB. Transposition of the Great Vessels

Transposition of the great vessels (TGV) is a congenital heart defect involving the "great vessels": the superior vena cava, inferior vena cava, pulmonary artery, pulmonary veins, and aorta. The ventricles and their respective arteries do not connect in the proper location due to a malrotation of the heart. Because of this rotation, the right (rather than left) ventricle leads to the aorta, and the left (rather than right) ventricle leads to the pulmonary artery and lungs (Figure 2-9).

Transposition of the great vessels is a congenital cyanotic heart defect in which the deoxygenated blood from the right heart is pumped into the aorta and delivered to the body, while the left heart pumps oxygenated blood to the pulmonary arteries and back to the lungs. There are 2 separate circulatory systems.

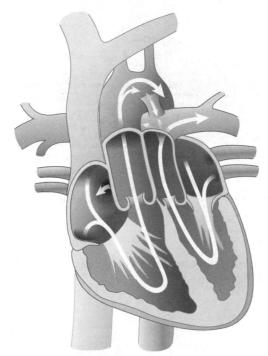

RA. Right atrium	SVC. Superior vena cava	TV. Tricuspid valve
RV. Right ventricle	IVC. Inferior vena cava	MV. Mitral valve
LA. Left atrium	MPA. Main pulmonary atery	AoV. Aortic valve
LV. Left ventricle	Ao. Aorta	ASD. Atrial septal defect
		PDA. Patent ductus arteriosis

FIGURE 2-9 Transposition of the Great Vessels (TGV). Used with permission from the Centers for Disease Control and Prevention.

Presentation

- Newborn with cyanosis, dyspnea, fatigue

Diagnosis

- Chest X-ray demonstrating an egg-shaped heart or the "egg-on-a-string sign," which demonstrates the abnormal structure caused by this condition
- Echocardiogram to evaluate structure

Treatment

- Surgical correction is the definitive treatment of the transposition.
- In newborns, prostaglandins must be given to keep the ductus arteriosus open. This allows the oxygenated and deoxygenated blood to mix.

BC. Patent Ductus Arteriosus

Patent ductus arteriosus (PDA) occurs when an infant's ductus arteriosus does not close after birth (Figure 2-10). The ductus arteriosus is located between the aorta and the pulmonary arteries. In utero, the ductus arteriosus is open, allowing for the passage of blood from the pulmonary artery to the aorta and the rest of the body. In utero, the blood bypasses the lungs, as the lungs are not used to oxygenate blood at this time. However, during the birth process, the ductus arteriosus should close, as blood will now need to pass through the lungs to become oxygenated. If this passage does not close, shunting and the mixing of oxygenated and deoxygenated blood can occur. Thus, deoxygenated blood will end up in the aorta to be sent to the rest of the body.

Presentation

- Hypoxia, cyanosis, dyspnea, growth restriction, tachycardia, cardiomegaly, widened pulse pressure

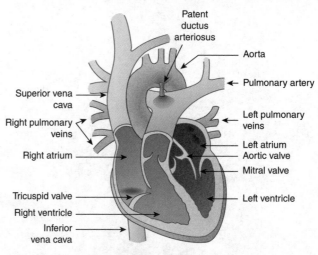

FIGURE 2-10 Patent Ductus arteriosus. Used with permission from the Centers for Disease Control and Prevention.

Physical Exam

■ Continuous machinery-like murmur

Diagnosis

■ Echocardiogram is used to evaluate for poor flow patterns.

Treatment

■ Mild patent ductus arteriosus can be closed with indomethacin.
■ Severe cases may require surgical repair of the PDA.
■ There are some conditions that require keeping the PDA open with prostaglandins such as misoprostol.

CLINICAL TIP
In order for children to survive transposition of the great vessels, the ductus arterious *must* remain open. Give misoprostol to keep the ductus patent.

C. GROWTH AND DEVELOPMENT

Milestones
Growth and development milestones are listed in Tables 2-2 through 2-11.

EXAM TIP
Tummy time starts at 1 month.

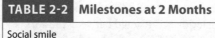

TABLE 2-2	Milestones at 2 Months
Social smile	
Localizes voices	
Localizes sounds	
Able to calm self	
Coos	
Tracks faces	
Fussy if not constantly entertained	
Can hold head up and push self up while lying on tummy	

TABLE 2-3	Milestones at 4 Months
Smiles spontaneously	
Social playing	
Expressive movements	
Babbling begins	
Differentiates cries	
Shows emotions	
Recognizes faces	
Holds head steady	
Pushes up to elbows on stomach	
May be able to roll from tummy to back	
Brings hands to mouth	
Reaches for toys	
Pushes legs down when feet are on hard surface	

TABLE 2-4	Milestones at 6 Months
Familiar facial recognition, differentiates between known individuals and strangers	
Plays with others	
Responds to emotions	
Recognizes self in mirror	
Differentiates sounds	
Responds to name	
Demonstrates joy and displeasure	
Rolls back to front and front to back	
Bounces and can support weight	
Rocking begins on all 4s	
Begins to string vowels together and may make consonant sounds	
Passes things from one hand to the other	
Starts to sit without support	

EXAM TIP
Infants start to eat solid foods at 6 months.

TABLE 2-5	Milestones at 9 Months
Stranger fear, clingy with familiar adults	
Has a favorite toy or item	
Understands "no"	
Babbles and can make some words understood; eg, mamama, bababa	
Points at items	
Looks for items that get hidden	
Puts things from hands into mouth, passes things from one hand to the other	
Can pull self up, crawl, and stand holding on to things	
Plays peek-a-boo	
Develops a pincher grasp	
Copies gestures	

TABLE 2-6	Milestones at 12 Months
Nervous with strangers, cries when parents leave	
Favorite items and people	
Shows fear	
Helps with dressing	
Understands and follows simple commands	
Says "mama" and "dada"	
Waves "bye-bye"	
Finds hidden items	
Explores and evaluates items	
Bangs things together	
Cruises	

EXAM TIP

General rule: First words, first birthday, first steps

TABLE 2-7	Milestones at 18 Months
Stranger anxiety	
Plays with others	
Shows affection	
Clings to caregiver in new situations	
Points to new, interesting things	
Says single words	
Understands "no"	
Points to wanted items	
Identifies common items	
Attracts the attention of others	
Can now follow more complex commands	
Walks unassisted, runs, climbs steps	
Undresses self	
Feeds self	

TABLE 2-8	Milestones at 2 Years
Demonstrates independence but copies others	
Engages in parallel play	
Defiant behavior, uses "no"	
Identifies items	
Constructs simple sentences	
Repeats words, can follow along in a book	
Imagination develops, plays make-believe	
Builds towers	
Kicks ball	

TABLE 2-9	Milestones at 3 Years
Affection for friends
Takes turns
Understands possessions
Demonstrates concern for others
Shows less stranger anxiety
Says simple words and phrases
Increased understanding of commands
Works moving parts, buttons
Can solve simple puzzles
Enjoys coloring
Can turn book pages and open doors and jars

TABLE 2-10	Milestones at 4 Years
Plays make-believe
Difficulty understanding difference between make-believe and real life
Plays house
Enjoys playing with other children
Memory increases, sings songs, remembers stories
Tells stories
Writing increases
Uses scissors
Understands the concept of time
States full name

TABLE 2-11	Milestones at 5 Years
Wants to emulate friends
Follows rules
Aware of gender
Able to differentiates between real life and make-believe
Likes to sing, dance, and act
Speaks more clearly, able to differentiate among tenses
Tells simple stories
Counting skills increase
More complex drawing
Fine motor skills increase, gross motor skills are well developed

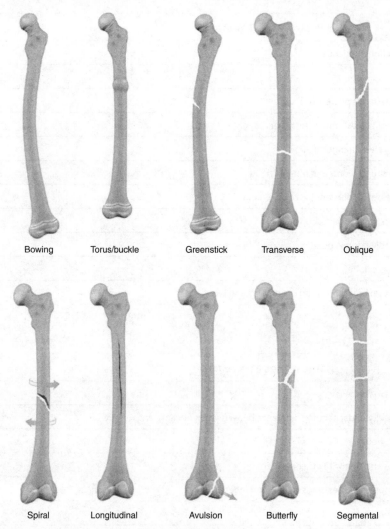

Bowing   Torus/buckle   Greenstick   Transverse   Oblique

Spiral   Longitudinal   Avulsion   Butterfly   Segmental

FIGURE 2-11 Different types of Fractures of Femur. Reproduced with permission from Elsayes KM, Oldham SA, eds. *Introduction to Diagnostic Radiology*. New York, NY: McGraw-Hill; 2015.

CLINICAL TIP
It is required by law to report known or suspected cases of child abuse. Your resources include child protective services agencies and the police.

CLINICAL TIP
You cannot be held liable for reporting suspected abuse or neglect.

CLINICAL AND EXAM TIP
• Look for injuries that do not appear to match the history given.
• Be on the lookout for chronic repetitive injuries.

D. ABUSE

Abuse is the physical, emotional, or verbal mistreatment of a child; for example, striking a child or not providing appropriate clothing. Neglect is a form of abuse in which the child's guardian is found to not be providing appropriate supervision or care; for example, medical or financial care.

The primary care nurse practitioner (NP) must be alert for signs such as inappropriately clothed children, injuries or wounds with questionable explanations, and recurring injuries that appear to be more than the result of a child being "accident prone." For example, certain types of fractures, such as greenstick or spiral, may be caused by abusive behaviors such as twisting motions (Figure 2-11).

E. VACCINES AT BIRTH AND THROUGHOUT CHILDHOOD

■ Vaccines are substances given to prevent disease.
■ They are typically given via injection but also occasionally through ingestion.
■ The majority of vaccines are given within the first 6 years of life (Figure 2-12).
■ The most common side effects of vaccine administration are site erythema and pain and low-grade fever.

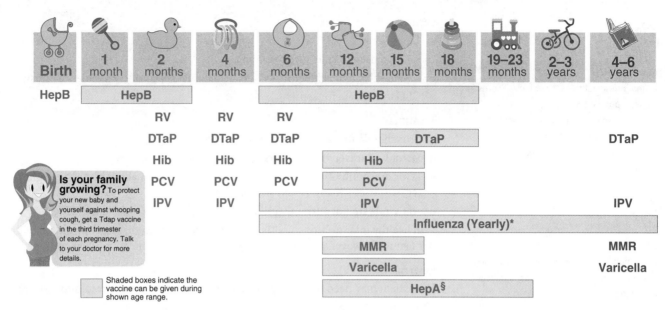

FIGURE 2-12 2015 Recommended immunizations for children from birth through 6 years old. Used with permission from the Centers for Disease Control and Prevention.

Occasionally parents or guardians choose to vaccinate their children on a modified schedule. The NP must assess the reasons why such a decision has been made and educate the parents or guardians about the risks and benefits of typical versus modified vaccination schedules.

F. RESPIRATORY SYNCYTIAL VIRUS AND BRONCHIOLITIS

Bronchiolitis, most commonly caused by respiratory syncytial virus (RSV), is an inflammation of the bronchioles at the terminal ends of the main bronchi. This is a condition common in children less than 2 years of age. Hospitalizations secondary to bronchiolitis peak between 2 and 6 months of age. Bronchiolitis is characterized by upper respiratory symptoms (eg, runny nose), followed by lower respiratory symptoms with inflammation (eg, wheezing, crackles). Edema and mucous build-up may cause an obstruction of the small airways and/or atelectasis.

Bronchiolitis Pathogens

- Bronchiolitis is usually caused by a virus, such as RSV, parainfluenza, rhinovirus (which is also causes the common cold), and influenza.
- In fall and winter, RSV is the most common cause.
- In spring and fall, parainfluenza is the most common cause.

Risk Factors for Severe Disease

- Premature birth
- Less than 12 weeks old
- Chronic pulmonary disease
- Congenital heart disease
- Immunodeficiency
- Neurological disease

Diagnosis

Clinical evaluation will likely elicit that the patient is experiencing decreased appetite, fatigue and lethargy, fever, and an increased respiratory rate. Retractions are a danger sign, and nasal flaring is a late and dangerous sign. Cough, congestion, runny nose, and fever may also be present.

EXAM TIP

The most common cause of bronchiolitis is respiratory syncytial virus (RSV), which causes approximately 70% of all cases.

Tests
- Chest X-ray
  - Often used to rule out pneumonia
  - Will show hyperinflation, peribronchial thickening, and possible atelectasis
- CBC to evaluate for sepsis

Treatment
- Bronchodilators, such as albuterol
- Steroids: intravenous (IV) solumedrol or oral prednisolone
- IV or oral antibiotics may be used if there is a question about bacterial origin (eg, suspicious X-ray, recent sick contact)
- Antivirals are not currently utilized for the treatment of bronchiolitis/RSV

In healthy infants, bronchiolitis is usually a self-limited disease. In children with risk factors, however, it may lead to respiratory failure, apnea, and dehydration.

Referral
The patient may need to be hospitalized if signs or symptoms of respiratory distress are noted.

G. CYSTIC FIBROSIS

Cystic fibrosis (CF) is diagnosed in the pediatric population. It is characterized by thick mucous and poor weight gain. This condition occurs in 1 in 3000 births. Chronic infections, difficulty breathing, clubbing of the fingers, and fat in the stool are also characteristic of the disease. Further information about cystic fibrosis can be found in Chapter 8.

H. FOODS

The developing child, from neonate to teenager, requires a large variety of nutritious foods. While it may be easier and cheaper for parents or guardians to provide non-nutritious foods, they must be counseled on the importance of proper diet for their children (Figures 2-13 and 2-14).

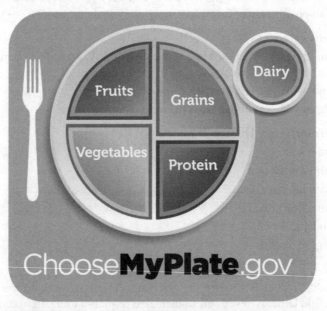

FIGURE 2-13 Used with permission of the United States Department of Agriculture.

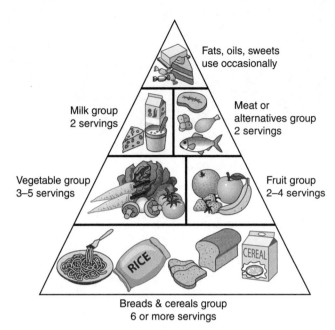

FIGURE 2-14 Used with permission from New York City Department of Education.

- Nonprocessed foods are better than processed foods.
- Whole-grain products have been demonstrated to be healthier than refined-grain products.
- Breastfeeding mothers need to increase their fluid intake and consume 1200-1500 calories per day.
- Vitamin D supplementation is also important while breastfeeding.

Solids

- Infants begin eating solid foods at 4 to 5 months of age, when they can hold their heads up by themselves.
- Foods such as 1 tablespoon of rice cereal with breast milk or formula is given.
- To be able to identify potential allergens, introduce only 1 new food every 4 days.
- Grains are introduced first, followed by vegetables, proteins, and fruit. Fruit is introduced last as it is sweet, and children will often prefer sweet foods over other types.

Exercise is an important aspect of developing childhood. The pediatric patient should be encouraged to participate in outdoor activities that are safe and burn calories.

CLINICAL TIP
Do not introduce honey until after age 1 year.

CLINICAL TIP
Do not introduce water until after age 18 months.

CLINICAL TIP
At age 1 year, stop formula and introduce whole milk.

3
Adolescent Medicine

GROWTH AND DEVELOPMENT

During adolescence the emphasis must change from monitoring development and growth to maintaining safety and fostering psychosocial development. Encouragement of the adolescent's spiritual and psychological development must be carefully monitored.

Puberty usually starts between the ages of 10 and 12 for females and between the ages of 11 and 13 for males. Puberty can be an emotionally traumatic time in the life of the adolescent, as many changes occur in the body and mind during this time. Parents often are also affected by the changes that occur in their children. Parents are often no longer the only source of input and guidance in their children's lives; rather, adolescents begin to rely more on the input of their friends. Table 3-1 lists the typical changes that occur in adolescence.

The Tanner stages describe the physical development of children and adolescents based on external primary and secondary sex characteristics, such as breast size, genitals, testicular volume, and the development of pubic hair. Tables 3-2 and 3-3 list the Tanner stages for females and males, respectively.

Drugs and Alcohol

During adolescence, young people may be exposed to substances both legal and illegal. The nurse practitioner must be sensitive but firm to keep the adolescent from harm. Table 3-4 lists some illegal and legal but dangerous substances adolescents may be exposed to. Table 3-5 describes the common effects of marijuana, cocaine, heroin, and ecstasy.

Safety

The most common cause of death among teenagers is trauma and accidents (Table 3-6). One factor is that many young people begin driving in adolescence. It is important for adolescents to understand the consequences of their actions.

TABLE 3-1	Typical Adolescent Changes
Mental • More independent • Full abstract thought • Sexuality contemplated	
Physical • Body develops (secondary sex characteristics)	

CLINICAL TIP
Females should demonstrate secondary sex characteristics by age 16. If not, an endocrine workup should be performed, including estrogen, thyroid-stimulating hormone (TSH), follicle-stimulating hormone (FSH), luteinizing hormone (LH), progesterone, and testosterone levels. A pelvic ultrasound should also be performed.

CLINICAL TIP
Cocaine can cause myocardial infarction, even in healthy young people.

CLINICAL TIP
The recreational use of legal drugs is more common than the use of illicit drugs.

TABLE 3-2 — Female Tanner Stages

TANNER STAGE	BREAST DEVELOPMENT	PUBIC HAIR DEVELOPMENT
1	Pre-puberty	No pubic hair
2	Breast buds	Few straight pubic hairs
3	Breast and areola grow as one	Darker and coarser hair
4	Breast and areola continue to grow; areola grows larger on top of breast	Darker and coarser hair that curls
5	Adult pattern	Adult pattern

TABLE 3-3 — Male Tanner Stages

TANNER STAGE	EXTERNAL GENITAL DEVELOPMENT	PUBIC HAIR DEVELOPMENT
1	Pre-puberty	No pubic hair
2	Testicular enlargement; rugae form	Few straight pubic hair
3	Penis gets longer	Darker and coarser hair
4	Penis gets wider	Darker and coarser hair that curls
5	Adult pattern	Adult pattern

TABLE 3-4 — Dangerous Substances Adolescents May Be Exposed To

ILLEGAL DRUGS	ABUSED LEGAL SUBSTANCES
Marijuana	"Bath salts"
Cocaine	Spray paint
Heroin	Aerosol sprays
Ecstasy	

TABLE 3-5 — Common Effects of Some Illegal Drugs

DRUG	SYMPTOMS	PHYSICAL FINDINGS
Marijuana	Euphoria, sedation, relaxation	Agitation, anxiety
Cocaine	Increased alertness, euphoria, rapid movements	Tachycardia (can cause myocardial infarction), insomnia, hypersomnia
Heroin	Sedation, decrease in pain, relaxation	Nausea, vomiting, abdominal cramps, agitation, rhinorrhea
Ecstasy	Euphoria, hallucination, decrease in anxiety	Tremors, anxiety, agitation

TABLE 3-6 — Causes of Death in Adolescence

The most common cause of death in the adolescent age group is trauma.

Suicide, drug abuse, and homicide are the next most common causes of adolescent death.

TABLE 3-7	Safe Sex Practices
Birth control: pills, shots, vaginal rings	
Condoms	
Abstinence	

Sexuality

Mid- to late adolescence can be a difficult stage because both males and females begin to contemplate their sexuality, and some struggle with their sexual identity. Some may begin to experiment with homosexuality or bisexuality. Teenagers must be encouraged to express their thoughts and feelings, and they must be taught safe sex practices (Table 3-7). Young people may face challenges as they navigate through this stage in terms of cultural or religious beliefs or fear that their choices will not be accepted by their peers or family.

Time must be spent discussing safe sex practices with the adolescent in a comfortable, safe environment. Appropriate use of contraceptives and prophylaxis against STDs, such as condoms, dental dams (latex used to cover the vaginal opening during oral sex), and other forms of safe sex, must be taught. Safe sex practices are usually discussed with adolescents in school-based health classes but the importance of such practices must be reinforced by the nurse practitioner. It is also important to provide counseling on the issue of unwanted pregnancy. The pros and cons of various birth control options are listed in Table 3-8.

Vaccines

The following vaccines should be administered to adolescents:

- Human papillomavirus (HPV)
- Meningococcal

    Ideal age for giving HPV is 11-26 and for Meningococcal is 11-18.

Screening Tests

The following screening tests should be done during adolescence:

- Height and weight
- Body mass index (BMI)
- Blood pressure
- Fasting lipid profile (if obese)
- Physical, emotional, and sexual abuse
- STD and HIV status if sexually active

CLINICAL TIP

Birth control does not equal safe sex.

Birth control *prevents pregnancy*.

Safe sex practices *prevent the transmission of sexually transmitted diseases*.

TABLE 3-8	The Pros and Cons of Different Types of Birth Control	
BIRTH CONTROL TYPE	**PROS**	**CONS**
Pill	Oral pill, easy to take	Needs to be taken at the same time every day
Vaginal ring	Insert and forget about it Local hormones	Must be inserted by the patient
Intradermal injection	Given every 3 months	Weight gain Unable to reverse effect if patient wishes to become pregnant during the 3-month period following injection
Intrauterine device (IUD)	Placed by obstetrician/gynecologist (OB/GYN) Lasts 5-10 years	Positioned inside the uterus

4

Geriatrics

ABUSE

- Laws concerning elder abuse (Table 4-1) vary from state to state, but the questions you will see on your examination will reflect the entire country. The questions will not be state specific because the examination is a national one.

- The nurse practitioner must keep a keen eye out for any signs of elder abuse. Elder abuse can be either mental or physical issue and can also encompass issues of medication neglect and neglect of proper care (Table 4-2).

- The nurse practitioner should be alert to any inconsistencies between patient and caregiver histories.

- A case of elder abuse is not defined by a specific age range. Rather, the term "elder abuse" is used to reflect the fragility and vulnerability of the patient. For example, a fully intact, self-supporting 80-year-old person living independently would not be considered a vulnerable elder on whose behalf you could take action without his or her consent. On the other hand, a 60-year-old person who has suffered a stroke and lives with diabetes, multiple sclerosis, or another chronic, debilitating illness would be a candidate for reporting suspected abuse because he or she is too fragile and vulnerable to take care of him- or herself independently.

- Healthcare providers do not need permission from the patient to report cases of suspected or known elder abuse to the authorities.

- In cases of suspected or known elder abuse, authorities such as an Adult Protective Services (APS) agency or the police should be contacted.

TABLE 4-1	Signs of Elder Abuse
Abnormal bruising
Poorly controlled chronic conditions
Fear when a family member or members are in the room

CLINICAL TIP
Do *not* write off bruising as "normal."

TABLE 4-2	Elder Abuse Encompasses Neglect
Not providing medications	
Not providing food	
Not providing adequate clothing	
Not providing other needed resources	

ACTINIC KERATOSIS

CLINICAL TIP
Actinic keratosis is a precursor to squamous cell carcinoma.

- Actinic keratosis consists of skin lesions that do not heal (Figure 4-1).
- Actinic keratosis occurs in elderly patients, most commonly in those with light or pale skin.
- The lesions appear as pink or red lesions and are located on areas of the body that are usually exposed to sun (eg, neck, face, arms).

Diagnosis

- Definitive diagnosis of actinic keratosis is by biopsy.

Treatment

- As a primary care nurse practitioner, your role is not to start treatment for actinic keratosis. Your role is to ensure the patient is referred to oncology for treatment and then to manage any comorbidities.
- The treatment for actinic keratosis is either fluorouracil (5FU) or imiquimod.
- Fluorouracil is a chemotherapy agent; in actinic keratosis, it is applied topically to the lesions.
- Imiquimod is a locally active immunostimulant that causes the painless sloughing off of the lesions.

ARCUS SENILIS

- In arcus senilis, a white ring forms around the cornea without vision changes being reported by the patient (Figure 4-2).

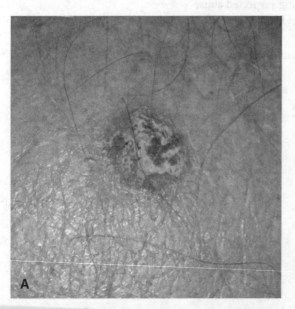
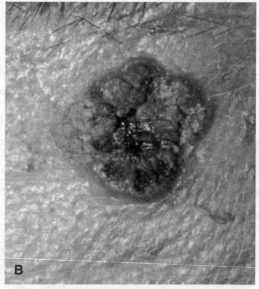

FIGURE 4-1 Examples of premalignant lesions: Actinic Keratoses. Reproduced with permission from Wolff K, Johnson R, Saavedra AP. eds. *Fitzpatrick's Color Atlas and Synopsis of Clinical Dermatology*, 7th ed. New York, NY: McGraw-Hill; 2013.

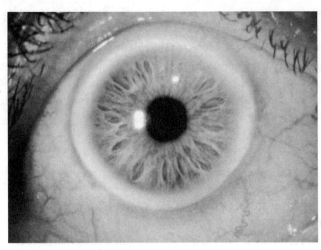

FIGURE 4-2 Arcus Senilis. The white ring at the edges of the cornea. Reproduced with permission from Riordan-Eva P, Cunningham ET, Jr. *Vaughan & Asbury's General Ophthalmology*, 18th ed. New York, NY: McGraw-Hill; 2011.

- The nurse practitioner must assess that no corneal changes have occurred.
- No treatment is needed for arcus senilis.
- Arcus senilis may be a sign of hyperlipidemia, but no therapy aside from the appropriate management of low-density lipoprotein (LDL) levels is necessary.

Diagnostic Tests
- Diagnosis is based on an assessment of the red reflex, conducted as part of a physical exam.
- The red reflex is assessed using an ophthalmoscope to examine the retina.

Eye Health in the Elderly
- Yearly ophthalmology exams for eye health (eg, glaucoma, cataracts, retinopathy) are indicated in the elderly population.
- Patients with diabetes mellitus type 2 should begin having dilated eye exams yearly upon diagnosis of their diabetes.

CLINICAL TIP
Make sure to check the red reflex.

NORMAL AGING

Normal Physical Exam
- **Head, eyes, ears, nose, and throat (HEENT)**: arcus senilis, sensorineural hearing loss
- **Skin**: seborrheic keratosis (wart-like skin lesions on the torso), lentigines (a benign process involving brown or tan macules on the hands and forearms)
- **Musculoskeletal**: decreased bone density (osteoporosis), decreased muscle mass, decreased fat mass, osteoarthritis
- **Cardiopulmonary**: mild changes to the shape, length, and thickness of the blood vessels; function of all receptions slows; lungs have decreased expiratory flow and elasticity
- **Abdominal**: stomach and intestinal flow decreases, as does absorption
- **Renal**: decreased kidney function and filtration speed
- **Endocrine**: decrease in hormone production and hormone sensitivity throughout the body

VACCINATIONS IN THE ELDERLY

The following vaccinations are offered in the elderly population:

- Tetanus: every 10 years; one of the vaccination should be tetanus, diphtheria, and pertussis (Tdap)
- Pneumococcal: Give 13-valent first, then 23 valent a year later once after age 65
- Herpes zoster: at age 60 or as soon as possible thereafter
- Influenza: yearly

SCREENING TESTS IN THE ELDERLY

- Dual energy X-ray absorptiometry (DEXA) scan to measure bone health in women at age 65; done every two years
- Abdominal aortic aneurysm (AAA) screening in men age 65 or over who were ever smokers; done only once

When to Stop Screening

The following screening exams should no longer be conducted after a certain age:

- Mammogram: age 75
- Pap smear: age 65
- Colonoscopy: about age 70

5
Cardiology

CHEST PAIN

Case 1

A 67-year-old female presents to the nurse practitioner having experienced 3 days of chest pain, which worsens with exertion. The patient has a past medical history of hypertension. Her vitals are as follows:

- Blood pressure (BP): 185/89 mm Hg
- Heart rate: 88 beats per minute
- Respiratory rate (RR): 18 breaths per minute
- Temperature: 36.2°C
- Pulse oximetry: 98% on room air

Which of the following interventions is appropriate?

A. Immediate transfer to emergency department (ED)
B. Electrocardiogram (EKG or ECG)
C. Nitroglycerin
D. Physician collaboration

Discussion

The correct answer is B. The primary step that a nurse practitioner must take is to establish a diagnosis. You do not need a physician to tell you to do an EKG on a patient experiencing chest pain. The EKG will not confirm all acute myocardial infarctions (MIs), but it is the most important first step in determining the origin of chest pain. Nitroglycerin is appropriate to administer if a cardiac origin is suspected, but the first priority in cases of chest pain is to determine if ST elevation is present on the EKG. Transferring the patient to the ED is critical, but it is not as important as first determining the presence of an infarction. There should be a provisional diagnosis prior to transferring care. Physician collaboration should be completed once there is a diagnosis.

Sources of Chest Pain

- A cardiac source of chest pain should be excluded first when a patient presents with chest pain.
- Do not forget that other organs, aside from the heart, can cause chest pain. The most common noncardiac origin of chest pain is the gastrointestinal (GI) tract.

TABLE 5-1	Sources of Chest Pain
Cardiac	
Respiratory	
Gastrointestinal	
Psychiatric	
Musculoskeletal	

- Ulcer and gastroesophageal reflux disease (GERD) are the 2 most common causes of noncardiac chest pain.
- Other body systems can also be a source of chest pain (Table 5-1).

Physical Exam

- A thorough heart, lung, peripheral vascular, and GI exam is important in the differential diagnosis of chest pain.
- There might not be anything present on the physical exam in myocardial infarction.
- The examination excludes a pulmonary origin (eg, wheezing, decreased breath sounds) for the chest pain and valvular heart disease.

Diagnostic Tests: EKG

- An EKG is the first step for diagnosing chest pain (Figure 5-1).
- ST segment elevation is defined as the elevation of 1 box in 2 contiguous leads; however, any elevation should be further evaluated.
- ST segment elevation means that the patient is having an acute myocardial infarction most of the time and that the patient should be transferred to the hospital for acute management such as percutaneous coronary intervention (PCI).
- ST segment depression is significant if a depression of 1 box is present in 2 contiguous leads. This means that the myocardium is becoming ischemic.

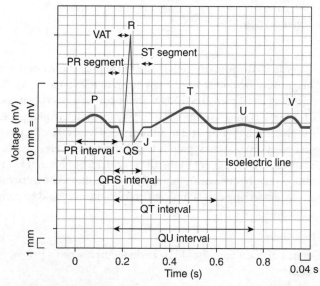

FIGURE 5-1 Normal EKG and labelling of normal waves. Reproduced with permission from Gomella LG, Haist SA: *Clinician's Pocket Reference: The Scut Monkey,* 11e. New York, NY: McGraw-Hill; 2007.

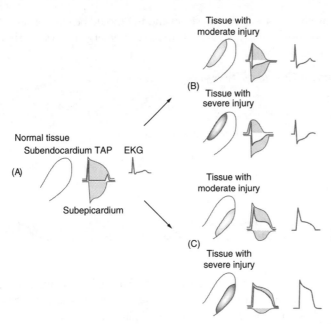

FIGURE 5-2 Patterns of myocardial tissue injury in ischemia. Reproduced with permission from Fuster V, Walsh RA, Harrington RA: *Hurst's The Heart*, 13e. New York, NY: McGraw-Hill; 2011.

■ T-wave inversions are significant when they are in 2 or more contiguous leads. They are also indicative of myocardium ischemia.

■ Q waves are an indication that the myocardium is dead. Q waves indicate a previous infarction.

Further Testing in Chest Pain

■ Pulse oximetry

■ Chest X-ray

■ Troponin and creatine kinase MB (CKMB) in the ED

■ Stress test if EKG is not diagnostic

Treatment

■ Treatment depends strongly on the most likely source of the chest pain (Table 5-2).

■ For cardiac-related chest pain, any patient with an abnormal EKG should be transferred to the ED to exclude acute coronary syndrome (ACS) and to ensure

TABLE 5-2	Treatment for Cardiac-Related Chest Pain
MEDICATION	EFFECT
Beta blocker	Slows heart rate Reduces metabolic demand
Nitroglycerin	Reduces preload and afterload
Angiotensin-converting enzyme (ACE) inhibitor/angiotensin receptor blocker (ARB)	Reduces vascular resistance Lowers BP
Aspirin	Decreases platelet aggregation
As a second antiplatelet medication: clopidogrel, prasugrel, or ticagrelor	P2Y12 platelet inhibitor
Low Molecular Weight Heparin	Used for ACS in the ED

CLINICAL TIP

- Oxygen does *not* lower the risk of mortality in MI.
- Assessment of the patient should precede the initiation of any treatment.
- Treatment with antiplatelet medications with Aspirin and one other antiplatelet medication is critical.

EXAM TIP

- On your exam, physician collaboration will most likely *not* be the correct answer.
- The purpose of the exam is to establish that the nurse practitioner can think for him- or herself.

CLINICAL TIP

After an acute event is over, proper follow-up and risk factor modification (eg, medication and diet compliance, smoking cessation, exercise programs) are key.

an MI has not occurred. The physician and ED should be made aware of the patient's condition, and, if applicable, the 911 or emergency system should be implemented.

Risk Factors for Coronary Disease

- Smoking
- Diabetes
- Family history of early-onset cardiac disease
- Obesity
- Hypertension
- Dyslipidemia

CONGESTIVE HEART FAILURE

Case 2

An 80-year-old male presents for follow-up after hospitalization for acute MI. He denies chest pain at present but states that his legs are swollen and that he now feels short of breath when he walks. His vitals are as follows:

- BP: 150/80 mm Hg
- HR: 76 beats per minute
- RR: 24 breaths per minute
- Temperature: 37°C

What is the most likely diagnosis?

A. Reocclusion of the vessel

B. GERD

C. Congestive heart failure (CHF)

D. Late-onset asthma

Discussion

The correct answer is C. The heart is a pump. When that pump fails, CHF occurs. Reocclusion of the vessel would most likely present similarly to the original acute MI (ie, with chest pain and other typical acute MI symptoms). GERD does not present predominantly with shortness of breath. Asthma does not begin suddenly at age 80. A patient with asthma would also present with obvious wheezing on examination.

CHF is a condition that results when the heart is unable to circulate blood appropriately. The different types of CHF are listed in Table 5-3.

TABLE 5-3	Types of Congestive Heart Failure
TYPE	DESCRIPTION
Right	Occurs as a results of left-sided failure Results in peripheral edema
Left	Heart loses pumping power Blood backs up into the liver and lungs Can be either systolic or diastolic
Systolic	Heart loses the ability to contract Low ejection fraction (EF) Loss of efficacy in pumping action
Diastolic Dysfunction	Heart loses its ability to relax Normal EF Heart cannot fully fill with blood between beats

Physical Exam

- Heart and lung exam is vital
- Assess for abnormal heart sounds such as S3 or S4
- Lung sounds: rales (crackles that does not clear with coughing), wheezing
- Peripheral vascular exam: pulses, edema, skin color

Diagnostic Tests

- An echocardiogram is indispensable to establish EF. A normal EF is 55-70%.

Treatment

- Treatment is based on the type and degree of CHF.
- Treatment begins upon diagnosis.
- Staples of treatment include beta blockers and ACE inhibitors or ARBs (Table 5-4).
- A left ventricular assist device (LVAD) may be used if the patient is still symptomatic after maximal medical therapy. The LVAD is a bridge to cardiac transplantation..
- Dietary modifications (low salt, fat, and cholesterol intake) and gentle exercise are beneficial.

Treatment for Systolic Dysfunction

- Start with an ACE inhibitor such as enalapril, ramipril, or lisinopril.
- The benefit of ACE inhibitors in systolic dysfunction is a class effect, so any ACE inhibitor is correct.
- ARBs are nearly as effective as ACE inhibitors, but if both ACE inhibitors and ARBs are possible, choose the ACE inhibitor.
- Some, but not all, beta blockers also lower mortality risk in systolic dysfunction.
  - The beta blockers effective in systolic dysfunction are carvedilol, metoprolol, and bisoprolol.
- Spironolactone and eplerenone inhibit the renin-angiotensin-aldosterone system and lower mortality risk.
- Although diuretics and digoxin decrease symptoms, they do not lower mortality risk.

Treatment for Diastolic Dysfunction

- No medication has clearly been proven to lower mortality risk in diastolic dysfunction.
- Beta blockers and diuretics are used routinely.

Adverse Effects of Treatment

- ACE inhibitors: cough, hyperkalemia
- ARBs: hyperkalemia
- Spironolactone: hyperkalemia, anti-androgenic effects (eg, gynecomastia)

TABLE 5-4	Medications for Congestive Heart Failure
MEDICATION	EFFECT
ACE inhibitor, beta blocker, spironolactone	Lowers mortality Eplerenone is used when gynecomastia occurs from the use of spironolactone
Ivabradine	Sodium channel blocker at the sinoatrial (SA) node When added to a beta blocker, lowers mortality
Sacubitril	When added to an ARB, lowers mortality Neprilysin inhibitor
Milrinone, dobutamine (home infusions)	Rarely ever needed as inotropes. A bridge to cardiac transplantation

TABLE 5-5	Common Causes of and Comorbidities with Peripheral Artery Disease
Diabetes	
Dyslipidemia	
Hypertension	
Smoking	

EXAM TIP
- Remember extra heart sounds: S3 with CHF and S4 with hypertension.
- Observe for weight gain.

CLINICAL TIP

Pain is associated more often with arterial disease than venous disease.

CLINICAL TIP

Cold limb with loss of blood supply = acute arterial embolus.

Comorbidities

- The comorbidities with CHF are similar to those with chest pain.

PERIPHERAL ARTERY DISEASE

- Peripheral artery disease (PAD) is a buildup of atherosclerotic plaque in the vessels of the legs. Table 5-5 lists common causes of PAD.
- This buildup is similar to that found in coronary and cerebral vessels and can cause a cerebrovascular accident (CVA) or MI.
- Look for pain in the legs on exertion (eg, walking) that improves with rest.

Physical Exam
- Diagnosis of PAD is difficult by physical exam alone.
- With PAD, there is a progressive loss of hair to the distal extremities; a glossy appearance appears and the distal pulses starts to become weak.
- Peripheral venous disease presents with chronic swelling. The skin may appear to be stretched. Severe swelling may result in weeping (yellowish discharge from the skin).

Diagnostic Tests

The ankle-brachial index (ABI) compares the patient's blood pressure in the lower extremities to the blood pressure in the upper extremities:

- If the lower-extremity blood pressure is 10% less than that in the upper extremities, there is a blockage.
- The ABI is used only for arterial disease, not venous disease.
- An ABI of < 0.9 is abnormal.
- An ABI of < 0.5 indicates a severe blockage.
- ABI = systolic leg BP ÷ systolic arm BP

An ultrasound of the artery determines the location and degree of stenosis in the vessel.

Treatment

Treatments for PAD include the following:

- Aspirin
- Clopidogrel
- Cilostazol
- Lifestyle modifications: glucose control, blood pressure control, smoking cessation
- ACE inhibitors are the best blood pressure medications in PAD

HYPERTENSION

Case 3

A 65-year-old female presents to the office with headache and slight lightheadedness. Upon assessment, the nurse practitioner finds that the patient's blood pressure is 150/100 mm Hg. The physical exam is otherwise normal. The patient admits to having just run to the office because she was late. The nurse practitioner re-evaluates the patient's blood pressure and obtains a reading of 140/86 mm Hg. The patient states that she now has no headache.

What is the appropriate first step of treatment?
A. Start lisinopril/hydrochlorothiazide (HCTZ) daily
B. Lifestyle modifications: decrease salt in the diet, lose weight
C. Start metoprolol
D. Send the patient to the ED

Discussion

The correct answer is B. This patient does not fit the definition of hypertension. In those above the age of 60, the cutoff for a diagnosis of hypertension is a blood pressure reading of over 150/90 mm Hg. Lifestyle modifications, such as decreasing salt in the diet, increasing exercise, and especially losing weight, are good measures for anyone. The initial choice of therapy for hypertension is either a thiazide diuretic, an ACE inhibitor, an ARB, or a calcium channel blocker. Lisinopril in combination with HCTZ are warranted only in cases in which blood pressure does not decrease after a course of monotherapy. Metoprolol is not a usual first-line medication unless there is also chest pain, palpitations, or similar symptoms presenting concurrently. This patient meets no criteria for ED transfer because she is asymptomatic.

Definition of Hypertension
- Generally, hypertension is defined as a blood pressure above 140/90 mm Hg.
- In those above the age of 60, hypertension is defined as blood pressure above 150/90 mm Hg.
- The cutoff for hypertension in diabetics is now the same as for the general population: 140/90 mm Hg.

Physical Exam
- Hypertension is known as the "silent killer" because of its lack of presenting signs or symptoms.
- The patient will often feel fine until his or her blood pressure is significantly elevated.
- The patient may complain of pressure in the head, pressure behind the eyes, chest pain, or shortness of breath.
- The symptoms associated with hypertension tend to be vague.

Causes of Hypertension
- Primary hypertension is without cause.
- Secondary hypertension results from renal or endocrine pathology (eg, renal artery stenosis, Cushing's syndrome, or other abnormalities of either pathway).

Diagnostic Tests
- Diagnosis of hypertension is clinical.
- The patient usually presents for a routine screening or nonrelated complaint, subsequently finding the blood pressure elevated.

Treatment
- Treatment is with either a thiazide diuretic, calcium channel blocker, ACE inhibitor, or ARB (Table 5-6).
- The specific drug class is not as important as getting the blood pressure under control.
- Beta blockers are more useful in coronary disease and CHF than in hypertension.
- If blood pressure is above 160/100 mm Hg, two different classes of medication will be used as part of initial therapy.

CLINICAL TIP
Hypertension is the most common cause of cardiovascular and neurologic events.

CLINICAL TIP
Hypertension is known as the "silent killer" because it causes damage to organs without signs or symptoms.

CLINICAL TIP
Different classes of medication work better in different ethnicities.

EXAM TIP
- First-line therapy in clinical practice is usually lifestyle modifications. This is often asked about on the exam.
- Be alert to the patient's stage of hypertension prior to determining treatment.

TABLE 5-6	Hypertension Medications	
CLASS	NAME	DESCRIPTION
Thiazide diuretic	Hydrochlorothiazide, chlorthalidone	Often used as first-line therapy
Loop diuretic	Furosemide	With CHF fluid overload
Beta adrenergic blocker (the "-lols")	Metoprolol, atenolol, labetolol	Often used after stroke or MI
Calcium channel blocker	Amlodipine, nifedipine, verapamil	Peripheral edema can occur with this class of medication
ACE inhibitor (the "-prils")	Lisinopril, enalapril, ramipril	Side effects include angioedema; dry, persistent cough; hyperkalemia
ARB	Valsartan, losartan, irbesartan, candesartan	Side effects include hyperkalemia

DEEP VEIN THROMBOSIS

Case 4

A 27-year-old female presents with a complaint of pain in her left calf. The patient's medication, medical, and surgical history is significant only for her use of an oral birth control medication. The patient states that she just returned from vacation.

Which test could be completed by the nurse practitioner to accurately diagnosis a deep vein thrombosis (DVT)?

A. Homan's sign
B. Arterial Doppler ultrasound
C. Venous Doppler ultrasound
D. Ankle-brachial index (ABI)

Discussion

The correct answer is A. Homan's sign involves the provider gently dorsiflexing the patient's foot. If positive, this will elicit pain in the calf, which may indicate DVT. This test is a good initial test as it involves a physical exam (always a good answer on the board exams).

An arterial Doppler ultrasound is performed for PAD. If the patient has good pulses, there is no reason to do an arterial Doppler. The ABI is also performed for PAD. A venous Doppler ultrasound is the most accurate test of DVT, but should not be the first test performed.

Warning Signs of DVT

- Cancer
- Joint replacement or fracture
- Hormonal birth control use in smokers
- Immobility
- Pregnancy
- Recent surgery

Primary Sources of DVT

- Antiphospholipid syndrome
- Protein C or S deficiency
- Factor V Leiden

Physical Exam

- DVT is a clot in the vein of an extremity (Figure 5-3).
- There may be pain, swelling, or erythema.
- The area usually feels warm and tender.

CLINICAL TIP

The major complication associated with DVT is the embolization (movement) of the clot to the lungs; this is called a pulmonary embolism.

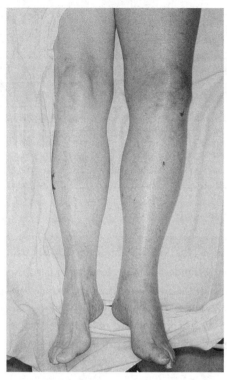

FIGURE 5-3 Appearance of an extremity affected by DVT. Reproduced with permission from Knoop KJ, Stack LB, Storrow AB: *The Atlas of Emergency Medicine*, 3e. New York, NY: McGraw-Hill; 2010. Photo contributor: Kevin J. Knoop, MD, MS.

Diagnostic Tests

- The key initial diagnostic test for DVT is Lower extremity doppler.

Treatment

- Treatment for DVT is anticoagulation (Table 5-7).
- Length of coagulation treatment depends on the site, the size of the clot or clots, how many clots are present, and the suspected cause.
- Patients are typically treated for 6 months.
- Lifelong therapy is indicated only if there are recurrent episodes of clotting.

Referral

- Hematology consultation is not needed in DVT patients.
- DVT therapy is the same regardless of the presence of protein C or S deficiency or factor V Leiden mutation.

CLINICAL TIP
Remember that anticoagulation will not dissolve the current clot, but rather will prevent future clots.

TABLE 5-7	Medications for Deep Vein Thrombosis
MEDICATION	DESCRIPTION
Enoxaparin	Patient must self-injection
Warfarin	Therapeutic at an international normalized ratio (INR) of 2-3
Dabigatran, rivaroxaban, apixaban, edoxaban	No INR monitoring Greater efficacy (less embolization) than warfarin Less bleeding as an adverse effect than warfarin
Fondaparinux	Factor Xa inhibitor Safe in heparin-induced thrombocytopenia (HIT)

TABLE 5-8	Hyperlipidemia Treatment
TREATMENT	**SIDE EFFECTS**
Lifestyle modification: diet and exercise	None
Niacin	Flushing
Fibrates: fenofibrate	Increased myalgias combine with statin
Statins: pravastatin, lovastatin, simvastatin, atorvastatin	Elevated liver function tests (LFTs) Rhabdomyolysis Myalgias

CLINICAL TIP
- High-density lipoprotein (HDL) is the "good" cholesterol.
- Low-density lipoprotein (LDL) is the "bad" cholesterol.

CLINICAL TIP
- Dyslipidemia is associated with cardiovascular and neurological conditions as well as pancreatitis.

CLINICAL TIP
Diet and exercise will always help.

EXAM TIP
Focus on diet and exercise.

DYSLIPIDEMIA

- Dyslipidemia, or hyperlipidemia, is an elevation of fats inside the blood.
- Fats are broken down into three categories: triglyceride, low-density lipoprotein (LDL), and very low-density lipoprotein (VLDL).
- There is usually no clinical presentation of dyslipidemia.
- Occasionally, primary dyslipidemia is caused by a protein or metabolism abnormality.

Diagnostic Tests
- Diagnosis is made via a lipid panel.
- A lipid panel is a *fasting* blood test.
- HDL monitoring adds little benefit.

Treatment
- First-line treatment is lifestyle modification (Table 5-8). Hyperlipidemia patients typically have a poor diet and exercise very little.
- Statin medications are always given for the following:
  - MI
  - ACS
  - Non-hemorrhagic stroke
  - Diabetes with LDL > 100 mg/dL
  - Carotid disease, aortic disease, or PAD with LDL > 70 mg/dL
  - Individuals with a 10-year risk of coronary disease > 7.5%

VALVULAR HEART DISEASES AND MURMURS

- Valvular heart diseases and murmurs occur when the valves at the junctures of the heart do not open and close as they are supposed to. This may be the result of a complication from disease (eg, rheumatic heart disease) or an anatomic abnormality (congenital or acquired).
- Systolic murmurs
  - Mitral regurgitation (MR)
  - Tricuspid regurgitation
  - Aortic stenosis (AS)
- Diastolic murmurs
  - Aortic regurgitation (AR)
  - Pulmonary regurgitation
  - Mitral stenosis (MS)

TABLE 5-9	Murmur Stages
Level 1	Audible only with special maneuvers
Level 2	Faint but audible with careful auscultation
Level 3	Readily audible, no thrill
Level 4	Audible with faint thrill (palpable murmur)
Level 5	Loudly audible, thrill, heard with stethoscope off the chest
Level 6	Loudly audible, thrill, can be heard without stethoscope

Presentation

- All valvular disease can present with shortness of breath and dyspnea on exertion.
- All valvular disease can lead to CHF.
- For regurgitant lesions, such AR and MR, the only symptom is the shortness of breath associated with CHF.
- With AS, the patient will experience chest pain from coronary disease and syncope.
- With MS, symptoms may also include atrial fibrillation (from a dilated atrium), dysphagia, and recurrent laryngeal nerve palsy (from a markedly enlarged left atrium).
- MS is the valve lesion most likely to be associated with stroke because of the enlarged left atrium and the high frequency of atrial fibrillation.
- Murmurs are classified into 6 stages (Table 5-9).

Diagnostic Tests

- Echo is the best initial test in all valvular disease. Although not often needed, cardiac catheterization is the most accurate test.
- The clinical exam will alert the nurse practitioner to the affected valve.
- The timing (systolic versus diastolic) will also provide clues as to which valve is affected and whether the valve is regurgitant or stenotic.
- An echocardiogram can also be conducted. This will clearly demonstrate the location and cause of the valvular abnormality.

Treatment

- Treatment depends on the stage of the murmur and whether the murmur is producing any clinical signs or symptoms (eg, feeling dizzy, syncope).
- AR and MR
  - Vasodilation with ACE inhibitors or ARBs
  - Surgical repair if the EF drops (< 55% in AR; < 60% in MR) or if the left ventricular end systolic diameter increases (> 55 mm in AR; > 40 mm in MR)
- AS
  - Replace valve if symptomatic
  - No medical therapy is effective
- MS
  - Dilate valve with balloon
  - Surgical replacement only if balloon dilation is ineffective

RHEUMATIC FEVER

Case 5

A 6-year-old male with a sore throat presented to the family practice nurse practitioner 2 days ago and was diagnosed with strep throat. He complains of worsening chest pain and body aches. The patient is febrile. The patient's mother states that he is pale and lethargic.

Which of the following is a potential diagnosis?

A. Myocardial infarction

B. Anxiety

C. Rheumatic fever

D. Pericardial effusion

CLINICAL TIP

The common bacteria in rheumatic fever is *Streptococcus pyogenes*.

CLINICAL TIP

Rheumatic fever can present after strep throat infection.

Discussion

The correct answer is C. The patient presents a clear-cut picture of rheumatic fever. Rheumatic fever occurs from streptococcal infections of the throat. Skin infections do not lead to rheumatic fever. Complaints of chest pain, fever, and arthralgias are common with rheumatic fever. Injection drug use leads to endocarditis, not rheumatic fever.

Physical Exam

- The patient will likely present with joint pain, chest pain, dyspnea, and fever.
- Rash may or may not be present.
- Signs of heart failure (eg, edema, rales in lung fields) may be present in cases of severe disease.

Diagnostic Tests

- A clinical exam is primary for diagnosis.
- A good history will allow the nurse practitioner to determine if risk factors are present.
- An echocardiogram may also be done to evaluate the heart tissue to see if vegetation is present on any valves.
- Antistreptolysin O (ASO) titers evaluate for the presence of a systemic streptococcal infection.

Rheumatic Fever Diagnostic Criteria

The Jones criteria are used to assist in the diagnosis of rheumatic fever. The major criteria are presented in Table 5-10, and the minor criteria are presented in Table 5-11.

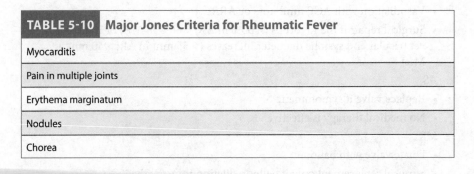

TABLE 5-10	Major Jones Criteria for Rheumatic Fever
Myocarditis	
Pain in multiple joints	
Erythema marginatum	
Nodules	
Chorea	

TABLE 5-11	Minor Jones Criteria for Rheumatic Fever
Fever	
Joint pain	
Elevated erythrocyte sedimentation rate (ESR) and/or C-reactive protein (CRP)	
Prolonged PR interval	

Treatment

- Treatment focuses on clearing the infection.
- Penicillin-based antibiotics work well (if the patient is not allergic).
  - If there is a penicillin allergy that causes only a rash, use a cephalosporin.
  - If there is a penicillin allergy that causes anaphylaxis, use vancomycin, linezolid, or daptomycin.
- Steroids and nonsteroidal anti-inflammatory drugs (NSAIDs) can be used to treat inflammation and pain.

6
Neurology

A. CEREBROVASCULAR ACCIDENT AND TRANSIENT ISCHEMIC ATTACK

Case 1

You are following up on a 70-year-old female who had been diagnosed with a possible cerebrovascular accident (CVA) or transient ischemic attack (TIA). The family describes the initial incident that brought the patient to the emergency department (ED) as a sudden loss of speech and motor function on the left side. The patient also had severely elevated blood pressure. She was admitted to the hospital and placed on aspirin and labetalol for blood pressure control. No thrombolytics were given, and no procedures were performed. The family states that all symptoms were gone within 24 hours.

Based on the likelihood that the patient had experienced a TIA, which of the following measures should be completed first?

A. Modification of lifestyle behaviors

B. Neurology referral

C. Test for diabetes

D. Test for dyslipidemia

Discussion

The correct answer is A. All answers are valid, but lifestyle modifications, such as quitting smoking, modifying diet, and getting more exercise, will decrease the likelihood that future events will occur. Testing for diabetes and cholesterol abnormalities are likely to occur as part of the follow-up appointment, but diagnostic tests are never the first-line answer. Referral to neurology should also occur, but again, is not the first-line answer.

Cerebrovascular Accident versus Transient Ischemic Attack

- CVA, or stroke, is a catastrophic deficit of neurological function that occurs via 1 of 2 mechanisms: thrombus or hemorrhage.
- TIAs are often referred to as "baby" strokes. During a TIA, symptoms of stroke present but reverse spontaneously within 24 hours.
- Signs of stroke occur on the opposite side of the body from the location of the clot or hemorrhage (ie, a right-sided clot will produce left-sided weakness and vice versa).

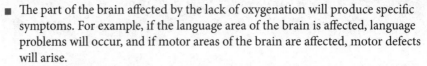

- The part of the brain affected by the lack of oxygenation will produce specific symptoms. For example, if the language area of the brain is affected, language problems will occur, and if motor areas of the brain are affected, motor defects will arise.
- Hemorrhagic stroke can occur as the result of an arteriovenous malformation (AVM). AVMs are tangles of defective blood vessels within the brain that have thin walls and can therefore weaken and burst.
- The type of hemorrhagic stroke, symptoms, and prognosis depend on the layers of brain tissue between which bleeding occurs.

Risk Factors for Stroke

- Hypertension
- Smoking
- Atrial fibrillation
- Diabetes

Treatment

Transient Ischemic Attack

- Aspirin
- If the patient is already on acetylsalicylic acid (aspirin), *switch* to clopidogrel or *add* dipyridamole.
- A statin
- Thrombolytics should *not* be given.

Ischemic Cerebrovascular Accident

- Within 3 (or 4.5) hours, the patient may be given tissue plasminogen activator (tPA) (referred to as a "clot buster") or undergo interventional neurologic procedures. The FDA approval is in all non-hemorhagic cases under 3 hours. In some circumstances it can be used up till 4.5 hours.
- Over 3 (or 4.5) hours, give aspirin.
- If the patient is already on aspirin, *switch* to clopidogrel **or** *add* dipyridamole.
- Within 6 hours, a catheter device may be used to physically remove the clot.

Hemorrhagic Cerebrovascular Accident

- In general, there is no specific therapy for hemorrhagic CVA.
- Do not confuse a hemorrhagic CVA with a subdural or epidural form of trauma.
  - Subdural or epidural forms of trauma can be treated surgically.
  - Hemorrhagic CVA is rarely, if ever, operated on.
- Emergency services should be contacted for any patient suspected of stroke.
- The collaborative physician should be called after making all efforts to stabilize the patient.

Diagnostic Tests

- A computerized tomography (CT) scan is always the first test to perform when stroke is suspected because you are looking for blood. You must exclude the presence of hemorrhage before any further therapy is indicated.
- A magnetic resonance imaging scan (MRI) is most accurate for diagnosing a nonhemorrhagic stroke.
- An echocardiogram is performed when any type of stroke is suspected in order to look for the source of the embolus.
- A carotid Doppler is performed because if there is 70-99% stenosis, carotid endarterectomy will be considered to prevent a subsequent stroke.
- A Holter monitor or telemetry is used to detect atrial fibrillation or flutter, which will require treatment with dabigatran, rivaroxaban, edoxaban, apixaban, or warfarin.

CLINICAL TIP
Early recognition and diagnosis are key to CVA and TIA prognosis.

CLINICAL TIP
CVA and TIA patients need to be cared for in the hospital setting.

- All patients with stroke or TIA and atrial fibrillation must receive long-term anticoagulation to prevent a subsequent stroke.
- Heparin is not needed for stroke prevention before giving oral anticoagulants.

B. PARKINSON'S DISEASE

■ Parkinson's disease is a degenerative disorder based in the central nervous system (CNS).

■ In Parkinson's disease, dopamine-producing cells in the substantia nigra (in the midbrain) die of unknown etiology.

■ Tremors, rigidity, decreased speed of movement, and gait abnormalities are characteristic (Table 6-1).

■ Age of onset is typically later in life, usually in the fifth decade.

■ Lewy body dementia is a type of dementia associated with Parkinson's disease.
  - Lewy bodies have been seen on autopsies of individuals with Parkinson's disease.
  - Lewy bodies are not used in the diagnosis of Parkinson's disease.

Diagnosis

■ Diagnosis is usually made by a neurologist.

■ A CT scan or MRI will show degeneration of the affected part of the brain; however, there is no specific diagnostic test for Parkinson's disease.

Treatment

■ Dopamine agents are the mainstay of treatment.

■ For mild disease consisting primarily of a resting tremor, amantadine or an anticholinergic agent, such as benztropine or trihexyphenidyl, is used.

■ Anticholinergic medications should be avoided in those over age 70 because they may lead to constipation, urinary retention, and dementia.

■ Direct dopamine agonists, such as pramipexole and ropinirole, are the standard of care as initial therapy in more severe disease. If these agents do not work, a combination of levodopa and carbidopa is used.

■ Patients not controlled with levodopa/carbidopa will have a catechol-O-methyl transferase (COMT) inhibitor, such as tolcapone or entacapone, added to the treatment regimen to extend the duration of the dopamine effect.

■ COMT inhibitors block the metabolism of levodopa and are used only in conjunction with levodopa/carbidopa.

■ As many as half of all elderly patients with severe Parkinson's disease will require such a large amount of medication that they will experience psychosis as a result of all the dopamine. If such a patient presents to you, do not stop the medications. Instead, add antipsychotic medications.

CLINICAL TIP
Ensure adherence to the treatment regimen and proper follow-up with neurology.

EXAM TIP
Bradykinesia, resting tremor, rigidity, and postural instability are hallmarks of Parkinson's disease.

TABLE 6-1	Symptoms of Parkinson's Disease
Tremor: usually occurs only in a single extremity at a time (eg, may appear in one extremity, stop in that extremity, and then appear in another extremity)	
Bradykinesia: slowing of motion, progressive throughout the course of disease	
Rigidity: stiffness and reduced range of motion	
Postural instability (late-stage symptom): decreased balance, increased incidence of falls	
Festination: shuffling gait, leaning forward while walking	
The "mask of Parkinson's disease": facial muscles become immobilized, resulting in a blank expression	

TABLE 6-2	Symptoms of Multiple Sclerosis
Changes in sensation
Vision problems
Difficulty swallowing
Acute or chronic pain
Depression, emotional liability
Sensitivity to temperature
Bowel or bladder problems

C. MULTIPLE SCLEROSIS

- Multiple sclerosis (MS) is an inflammatory disorder affecting the covering of the neurons in the CNS.
- MS can produce symptoms of motor, sensory, or visual disturbances (Table 6-2).

Diagnosis

- Diagnosis is usually made by a neurologist.
- An MRI is 95-98% sensitive and specific for the diagnosis of MS.
- An MRI will demonstrate the areas of neuronal demyelination (lesions or plaques).
- Rarely, analysis of cerebrospinal fluid from a lumbar puncture for oligoclonal bands is needed.

Treatment

- Treatment is typically initiated and maintained by a neurologist.
- Treatment is aimed at reducing the frequency, duration, and intensity of symptoms (Table 6-3).
- Acute episodes of neurological dysfunction are treated with high-dose glucocorticoids.
- To prevent symptom recurrence, immunosuppressive medications are used:
  - Beta interferon
  - Glatiramer
  - Mitoxantrone
  - Natalizumab (causes progressive multifocal leukoencephalopathy)
  - Fingolimod (the only oral drug currently available for MS)
  - Dalfampridine (increases walking speed)

CLINICAL TIP

Make sure your patients are compliant with their medication regimen to prevent an exacerbation of symptoms.

TABLE 6-3	Symtom-Specific Treatment for Multiple Sclerosis
MANIFESTATION	TREATMENT
Fatigue	Amantadine
Neurogenic bladder (atonic)	Urecholine
Spasticity	Baclofen, tizanidine
Urge incontinence	Oxybutynin, tolterodine

EXAM TIP

Early symptoms of MS can be vague; for example, blurry vision, numbness, and tingling.

D. MYASTHENIA GRAVIS

- Myasthenia gravis is a neurological condition caused by the loss of acetylcholine receptors at the neuromuscular junction interfering with nerve transmission, resulting in muscle weakness.

Signs and Symptoms of Myasthenia Gravis
- Fatigue (hallmark sign)
- Progressive muscle weakness with repetitive use
- Decrease in eye muscle and other facial functions
- Paralysis of respiratory muscles in acute, severe cases

Diagnosis
- Diagnosis is via bloodwork looking for acetylcholine receptor antibodies.
- Electromyogram (EMG) is the most accurate test for myasthenia gravis diagnosis.

CLINICAL TIP
There is a childhood form of myasthenia gravis: pediatric congenital myasthenia.

Medications
- Medications to inhibit acetylcholinesterase, such as pyridostigmine or neostigmine, will likely be prescribed by neurology.
- When chronic disease progresses to the point where it can no longer be controlled by medications, disease remission is induced by removing the thymus gland.
- In cases of acute, severe myasthenia crisis, treatment with intravenous (IV) immunoglobulin is initiated.

CLINICAL AND EXAM TIP
Myasthenia gravis involves the weakening of the voluntary muscles and eyelids.

E. TERTIARY SYPHILIS

- Late syphilis becomes neurosyphilis, which becomes problematic as it results in neurologic symptoms.

Signs and Symptoms of Tertiary Syphilis
- Gait abnormalities
- Vision disturbances
- Confusion or personality changes
- Depression
- Dementia
- Headache
- Memory problems
- Mood disturbances
- Bowel or bladder problems

CLINICAL TIP
Tertiary syphilis can be prevented by the proper treatment of primary or secondary syphilis.

Diagnosis
- Blood tests for syphilis include venereal disease research laboratory (VDRL), rapid plasma reagin (RPR), and fluorescent treponemal antibody absorption (FTA-ABS). FTA is 100% sensitive in the CSF.
- A cerebrospinal fluid (CSF) test may also be done. A negative FTA on CSF excludes neurosyphilis.

Treatment
- Penicillin is the treatment of choice for neurosyphilis; 3-4 million units of penicillin G every 4 hours for 10-14 days is prescribed.
- There is no effective substitute for penicillin in the treatment of neurosyphilis.

CLINICAL TIP
In cases of dementia, exclude neurosyphilis.

F. TRIGEMINAL NEURALGIA

- Trigeminal neuralgia is severe pain along the trigeminal nerve (cranial nerve V).
- The trigeminal nerve is entirely a sensory nerve of the face.
- The pain caused by trigeminal neuralgia can last from minutes to hours.
- The pain is described as a stabbing, electric-shock, or burning sensation.

Diagnosis

- Diagnosis is clinical by history and physical exam.
- Nothing will be visible on the physical exam.
- Pain may be produced by stimulating the trigeminal nerve.
- Nerve conduction studies are the most accurate diagnostic tests.
- An MRI may show a compressive lesion in some cases.

Treatment

- Carbamazepine is the first drug to try.
- Other anticonvulsants may also be used.
- Phenytoin, valproic acid, lamotrigine and gabapentin are examples of medications that are effective for both seizures and neuropathic pain, such as that caused by trigeminal neuralgia or peripheral neuropathy.
- Opioid analgesics and muscle relaxants may also be used for pain relief.
- If medications are ineffective, surgical decompression will be attempted.

G. SEIZURES

- Seizures are the result of abnormal signals sent from the brain that "short-circuit" normal neurological function.
- This "short-circuiting" results in anything from periods of somnolence (absence seizures), to single-extremity contractions (partial, or petit mal, seizures), to full-body convulsions (tonic-clonic, or grand mal, seizures).
- In a "simple" seizure, there is no loss of consciousness.
- In a "complex" seizure, there is loss of consciousness.
- To be considered as having epilepsy, a patient must have experienced more than 1 seizure with no identified underlying cause.
- Seizures resulting from sodium, glucose, or calcium disorders are *not* epilepsy.
- Seizures may or may not be preceded by an aura (abnormal sights, smells, or sensations).
- Focal, or partial, seizures occur in just one part of the body and involve a specific muscle group.
- Focal seizures may advance to generalized seizures.
- Generalized seizures involve loss of consciousness.

Types of Seizure

Table 6-4 lists the types of seizure.

After a Seizure

- After a seizure, the patient may be in a confused state called a postictal state.
- The altered mental status of the postictal state can last from a few minutes to several hours. It is unusual for the postictal state to last more than 24 hours.
- The patient will usually feel tired, confused, irrational, or combative and may complain of a headache.
- Status epilepticus is a generalized tonic-clonic seizure lasting more than 5 minutes or more than 1 seizure occurring within a 5-minute period without the patient returning to normal between them. The seizure or seizures are persistent, without allowing the muscles to relax. Status epilepticus is a life-threatening emergency.

TABLE 6-4	Types of Seizure
SEIZURE TYPE	DESCRIPTION
Tonic-clonic	Contraction and relaxation of the limbs in a cyclic fashion Can also cause contraction of the respiratory muscles
Clonic	Shaking of the limbs
Tonic	Persistent contraction of muscles Can affect the respiratory muscles
Myoclonic	Local or generalized muscle spasms
Absence	Eyelid twitching Patient appears to be in a daze
Atonic	Loss of muscle function

Causes of Seizures

Causes of seizure include the following:

- Hypoglycemia
- Hypocalcemia
- Hypoxia
- High or low sodium
- Head trauma
- Intracranial lesion
- Liver or renal failure

Diagnosis

- The diagnosis of epilepsy is usually made by a neurologist.
- However, patients usually present to the primary care nurse practitioner or ED after experiencing their first episode.

Diagnostic Tests

- All patients with a new onset of seizure should have their glucose, calcium, oxygen, sodium, and magnesium levels tested.
- A brain CT or MRI should be performed.
- If all test results are normal, an electroencephalogram (EEG) should be performed.
  - An EEG monitors brain waves.
  - An EEG is performed only if all other test results are normal.

Treatment

- Anticonvulsant therapy is usually initiated by the neurologist.
- The primary care nurse practitioner's role is to ensure the patient is compliant with their medication regimen, monitor medication levels in conjunction with the neurologist.
- Acute status epilepticus is treated with IV medications in sequence if the seizure does not stop:
  - A benzodiazepine (eg, lorazepam)
  - Fosphenytoin
  - Phenobarbital
  - General anesthesia (eg, propofol, midazolam)

CLINICAL TIP

Ensuring patient adherence to medication is the best way to prevent breakthrough seizures.

CLINICAL TIP

Be aware that states have different laws about allowing patients to drive after experiencing a seizure.

EXAM TIP

- Safety is the #1 priority in patients with seizure.
- For exam questions about seizure diagnosis, focus on the type of convulsion, and whether the whole body or only part of the body is involved.

■ Chronic anti-epileptic drugs (AEDs) are used for long-term epileptic seizure control.

- Do *not* treat a single seizure with an AED.
- There is no clear first choice for long-term AED treatment.
- Phenytoin, valproic acid, levetiracetam, carbamazepine, and lamotrigine, among others, are all possible first-line choices.

Who Should Be Treated with a Long-Term AED After Just One Seizure?

■ Patients presenting with status epilepticus

■ Patients in whom the source of seizure cannot be corrected, such as an intracranial lesion

■ Patients in whom the EEG is abnormal

■ Patients with a strong family history of recurrent seizures

7

Gastroenterology

A. GASTRITIS

Gastritis is the irritation and erosion of the lining of the stomach. The causes of gastritis are listed in Table 7-1.

Gastritis is usually described as a burning or gnawing sensation in the epigastric area or left upper quadrant (LUQ). This may be associated with gastrointestinal bleeding.

Treatment

Gastritis is treated by removing the offending agent (ie, stopping or decreasing alcohol or NSAID consumption). Medications are used with the goal of decreasing the acidity of the stomach or providing protection of the stomach tissue from the acidic environment of the stomach (Table 7-2).

Diagnosis

There is no way to make the diagnosis of gastritis without endoscopy. You cannot tell ulcer disease from gastritis without endoscopy. Serologic testing for *Helicobacter* cannot tell you whether the patient has gastritis, gastric ulcer, duodenal ulcer, or nonulcer dyspepsia.

Referral

Referral to gastroenterology (GI) should be completed if the patient is under age 45-55 years and fails a trial of oral medications and dietary and lifestyle modifications. Patients with epigastric pain above the age of 45-55 should undergo endoscopy.

Make sure to tell your patients that dietary and lifestyle modifications and taking medication will do nothing if they are smoking a pack a day or drinking alcohol.

DANGER SIGNS

Each of the following warrants immediate endoscopy:
- Blood in stool
- Weight loss
- Dysphagia
- Odynophagia
- Anemia

CLINICAL TIP

PPIs such as pantoprozole (Protonix), esomeprazole (Nexium), or omeprazole (Prilosec) are usually given first. PPIs are effective in 95% of patients. H2 blockers such as ranitidine (Zantac), famotidine (Pepcid), nizatidine, and cimetidine are effective in 70% of patients.

TABLE 7-1	Causes of Gastritis
Nonsteroidal anti-inflammatory drugs (NSAIDs)	
Alcohol	
Helicobacter Pylori	
Pernicious anemia (B12 deficiency)	

TABLE 7-2	Medications for Gastritis	
CLASS	NAME	EFFECT
Histamine H2 receptor antagonist (H2 blocker)	Famotidine (Pepcid), ranitidine (Zantac)	Acid reducer
Proton pump inhibitor (PPI)	Pantoprozole (Protonix), esomeprazole (Nexium), omeprazole (Prilosec)	Acid reducer
Other	Carafate	Stomach liner

CLINICAL TIP
Medications such as calcium channel blockers can cause GERD, as well as hernias, to occur.

CLINICAL TIP
GERD is a cause of chronic cough in all ages.

CLINICAL TIP
If blood is present, GI referral is warranted.

B. GASTROESOPHAGEAL REFLUX DISEASE

Gastroesophageal reflux disease (GERD) occurs when the acidic contents of the stomach are introduced into the esophagus. This is usually related to an inappropriate relaxation of the esophageal sphincter.

Presentation

Patients have burning epigastric pain. Some have a bad taste in their mouth, cough, and hoarseness. In pediatrics, this can also present as postprandial vomiting (vomiting after eating) or chronic cough. Exacerbating factors are presented in Table 7-3.

Diagnosis

Diagnosis includes a careful history and physical. Tests that may be performed include response to PPIs (this is the usual test), esophagogastroduodenoscopy (EGD) (in which a camera is passed via fiber-optic scope by the gastroenterologist), and a 24-hour esophageal pH monitor in equivocal cases.

Treatment

Medications for GERD are similar to those for gastritis (Table 7-4).
    If medications are ineffective, surgical tightening of the sphincter is performed.

Referral

If there is no response to PPIs, GI consultation is warranted for a 24-hour pH monitor and possible endoscopy. If PPIs are ineffective, surgical or endoscopic procedures are needed to tighten the lower esophageal sphincter.

TABLE 7-3	Exacerbating Factors
Hiatal hernia	
Obesity	
Alcohol, nicotine, chocolate, peppermint	
Eating in bed	
Pathology such as scleroderma	

TABLE 7-4	Medications for GERD	
CLASS	NAME	EFFECT
H2 blocker	Famotidine (Pepcid), ranitidine (Zantac)	Acid reducer
PPI	Pantoprozole (Protonix), Esomeprazole (Nexium), omeprazole (Prilosec)	Acid reducer

C. HEPATITIS

Hepatitis is the acute or chronic inflammation of the liver. It may have sexually transmitted disease (STD) or non-STD origins (Table 7-5).

Overuse or abuse of acetaminophen (eg, Tylenol) can also cause inflammation of the liver (noninfectious hepatitis).

Presentation

There are usually no symptoms of chronic hepatitis B or C. With acute hepatitis, the patient is markedly jaundiced with malaise, fatigue, and myalgias.

Acute hepatitis A usually presents with jaundice, nausea, vomiting, diarrhea, abdominal pain, or cramping. All forms of acute hepatitis are associated with dark urine because of direct conjugated bilirubin going into the urine. Weight loss is common in all forms of acute hepatitis because of anorexia.

Diagnosis

All forms of acute hepatitis are associated with the following:

- Elevated direct bilirubin
- Elevated alanine transaminase (ALT)
- Bilirubin on urinalysis

Albumin and prothrombin time should be normal. Specific diagnostic tests are presented in Table 7-6.

TABLE 7-5	Common Sources of Hepatitis Infection
Sexual intercourse	
Contaminated food or water (hepatitis A)	
Injection drug use (hepatitis B and C)	
Hepatitis D: injection drug use only if hepatitis B present	
Hepatitis E: pregnant women, usually of southeast Asian origin	
No identified risk in 30-40%	

TABLE 7-6	Specific Diagnostic Tests for Hepatitis
HEPATITIS TYPE	**DIAGNOSTIC TEST**
A, D, E	Immunoglobulin M (IgM) acutely Immunoglobulin G (IgG) upon resolution
C	Antibody test first Polymerase chain reaction (PCR) RNA viral load to confirm level of activity Genotype to predict response
Acute B	Surface antigen (SAg) E antigen (eAg) Core antibody IgM
Chronic B	Persistence of surface antigen > 6 months eAg either positive or negative Core antibody IgG
Vaccine to B	Only surface antibody positive
Resolved (past) B	Surface antibody Core antibody IgG

Treatment

Hepatitis A usually resolves on its own. Hepatitis B and C patients should be referred to GI for further management. The only form of acute hepatitis that is treatable is hepatitis C. There are multiple options for hepatitis C with equal efficacy. The choice of the individual drug is beyond the scope of your examination. For acute hepatitis C, give ledipasvir and sofosbuvir. This treatment is also used for chronic hepatitis C.

Chronic hepatitis B is treated with one of the following, although it is not clear which has the best efficacy:

- Lamivudine
- Entecavir
- Adefovir
- Tenofovir
- Telbivudine

Prevention

Hepatitis A and B vaccinations are part of the normal vaccine schedule for newborns. The adult patient should have occasional monitoring of titers for hepatitis B to assess immunity, especially if the patient is high-risk (eg, men who have sex with men, those who are HIV positive, anyone planning upcoming travel). All patients born between 1945 and 1965 should be tested for hepatitis C.

D. PANCREATITIS

Pancreatitis is the inflammation of the pancreas. It is not associated with diabetes. Table 7-7 lists the common causes of pancreatitis.

Pancreatitis usually presents as sudden epigastric pain radiating to the back. Nausea and vomiting occur frequently. The patient will usually be unable to tolerate food.

Diagnosis

Ultrasound and computerized tomography (CT) scan will demonstrate an inflamed pancreas. This imaging will demonstrate gallstones or gallbladder disease if present. In the blood work, amylase and lipase (pancreatic enzymes) will be elevated. Significantly elevated triglycerides may also be present.

The CT scan does three things:

1. Diagnoses the presence of acute pancreatitis
2. Determines the presence of correctable etiologies such as stones, strictures, tumor, or obstruction
3. Finds necrosis if present; if > 30% of the pancreas is necrotic, a biopsy (removal of tissue for microscopic evaluation) will be needed to exclude infection, and the patient will need antibiotic treatment with imipenem.

Treatment

The patient will likely require admission to the hospital, so an emergency department (ED) referral should be made. GI referral will also typically be ordered for management. The patient should be designated nothing by mouth (NPO) to give the pancreas a rest. The single most important management in severe acute pancreatitis is high-volume intravenous fluids. Pain medication usually includes a narcotic.

TABLE 7-7	Common Causes of Pancreatitis
Gallstones	
Alcohol	
Hypertriglyceridemia	
Trauma	

E. DIARRHEA: INFECTIOUS VERSUS NONINFECTIOUS

Diarrhea is three or more loose, watery stools within 24 hours.

The patient should always be assessed for localized abdominal pain, fever, and blood in stool. A good history is very important; ensure to ask about recent travel, new foods introduced to the diet, new medications taken (eg, antibiotics), and so on. Blood in the stool and fever usually represent infectious diarrhea. If antibiotics have been used recently, especially clindamycin, *C. difficile* infection is likely.

DANGER SIGNS
- Blood in stool
- Hypotension
- Fever

F(A). IRRITABLE BOWEL DISEASE: ULCERATIVE COLITIS AND CROHN'S DISEASE

Ulcerative colitis (UC) is the inflammation and ulceration of the large intestine. Crohn's disease is the inflammation and ulceration of the entire intestinal tract. Both conditions are autoimmune diseases and classified under the umbrella term of inflammatory bowel disease (IBD).

Irritable bowel disease (IBD) can also be related to inflammation outside the intestinal tract. IBD may affect the eyes, skin, joints, and liver and can cause colon cancer. Genetics also have a role in the progression of IBD.

CLINICAL TIP
UC and Crohn's disease differ in that UC is confined to the large intestine, whereas Crohn's disease may affect the entire GI tract.

Presentation

The patient will present with diarrhea that may be bloody or mucous stained. Weight loss, oral food intolerance, and blood on rectal exam may also be present.

Diagnosis

Blood will be noted on rectal exam. The final diagnosis is made by a gastroenterologist via endoscopy. Blood panels for inflammation and inflammatory bowel disorders should also be ordered. Autoimmune panels, ESR and CRP should also be ordered.

Treatment

Acute exacerbations of IBD are treated with steroids (glucocorticoids). Budesonide is particularly useful in IBD because it predominantly acts locally and is detoxified in the liver, thereby decreasing the frequency of systemic adverse effects. Medications for IBD are given in Table 7-8.

Biological Therapy

Tumor Necrosis Factor Inhibitors

Tumor necrosis factor (TNF) inhibitors are critical, must-know drugs. They are used to close up a fistula, which is an abnormal connection between the bowel and another organ such as the bladder, vagina, or skin. Fistulae occur only with Crohn's disease: the bowel melts a hole through organs it is touching. This leads to defecation through the anterior abdomen. Bowel-to-bowel loop fistulae are common as well.

TABLE 7-8	Medications for Irritable Bowel Disease
CLASS	NAME
5-ASA derivative	Mesalazine
Biological therapy	Infliximab, adalimumab
Steroid	Prednisone
Immunosuppressant	Azathioprine, 6-mercaptopurine
Probiotic	

TNF inhibitors are associated with the reactivation of tuberculosis (TB). You will definitely need to know how to perform purified protein derivative (PPD) and only one interferon gamma release assay (IGRA) tests. One of these is performed prior to the start of therapy. You must start isoniazid if one of these TB tests is positive. You can still give the TNF inhibitor to close the fistula, but the isoniazid must be started as well.

Surgery

Surgical removal of the colon cures ulcerative colitis but is a last resort. Surgery is less effective for Crohn's disease as it can recur at the site of anastomosis (connection). Surgery is used in Crohn's disease to unblock obstructions.

Screening for Colon Cancer

Both UC and Crohn's disease are associated with the development of colon cancer. Colonoscopy is performed if IBD of either type has involved the colon for more than 8 to 10 years. Crohn's disease involves the colon in half of all Crohn's patients. Colonoscopy must be performed in all IBD patients with colonic involvement every 1-2 years with biopsy even if there are no symptoms. The nurse practitioner (NP) must know that this needs to be done because the gastroenterologist cannot refer patients to him- or herself out of your practice. You must identify them.

Referral

The patient should be referred to gastroenterology for final diagnosis. Endoscopy and colonoscopy should be completed to determine the extent of disease.

EXAM TIP
Know the difference between UC and Crohn's disease.

CLINICAL TIP
Colon cancer should be ruled out.

F(B). IRRITABLE BOWEL SYNDROME

Irritable bowel syndrome (IBS) is a chronic cluster of intermittent abdominal discomfort, bloating, and change in bowel habits (diarrhea or constipation). There is no clear cause, but there is an association with depression. IBS is divided into three categories (Table 7-9).

Prior to diagnosis, organic diseases such as celiac disease, UC, Crohn's disease, and colon cancer must first be ruled out.

Presentation

Diagnosis is usually clinical. The patient usually reports abdominal discomfort, intermittent diarrhea, or constipation. There may also be bloating or a sensation of incomplete bowel evacuation. IBS is a pain syndrome: there is pain with diarrhea, constipation, or both.

There is no known cause of IBS, and there are no lab examinations to conclusively establish a diagnosis of IBS. Gastroenterology consultations can be obtained to rule out other pathology. Endoscopy, CT, and stool studies will all be normal.

Treatment

Medications for IBS are given in Table 7-10, and therapy options are given in Table 7-11. All forms of irritable bowel syndrome benefit from fiber.

TABLE 7-9	IBS Categories
IBS-D (diarrhea)	
IBS-C (constipation)	
IBC-A (alternating diarrhea and constipation)	

TABLE 7-10	Medications for IBS		
IBS TYPE	CLASS	NAME	EFFECT
All types	Anxiolytic	Tricyclic antidepressants	
IBS-D	Antispasmotic	Dicyclomine, hyoscyamine	Relaxes the bowel wall
	Probiotic		
IBS-C	Laxative	Linaclotide, Lubiprostone	

TABLE 7-11	Therapy Options For IBS
Cognitive behavioral therapy (CBT)	
Hypnosis	
Immersion therapy (exposing the patient to a known stressor in a controlled environment)	

G. COLON CANCER

Colon cancer is a collection of abnormal cells in one portion of the colon. Family history is the most important risk factor. Colon cancer in first-degree relatives (parents or siblings) increases the risk in the patient. Colon cancer in any first-degree relative changes the urgency of screening to start at age 40 rather than 50. Smoking and alcohol use each may increase the risk of colon cancer, but such use does not change the recommendation for colonoscopy screening to start at age 50.

Presentation

The patient may have mild abdominal cramping, blood in the stool, and weight loss. Such symptoms are usually indicative of advanced cancer, as symptoms will not appear until the tumor is large enough to cause them.

Diagnosis

The diagnosis is made via colonoscopy. A biopsy will also be taken.

Treatment

The patient should be placed under the care of gastroenterology and hematology/oncology immediately. Surgical resection (removal) and chemotherapy and/or radiation therapy should be guided by these specialists.

Screening Asymptomatic Patients

Screening is the single most frequently asked colon cancer question in your examination. Routine screening starts at age 50 in the general population. If the patient has a first-degree relative with colon cancer, start screening at age 40, or 10 years earlier than the age at which the family member was diagnosed, whichever is earlier.

Colonoscopy is far better than sigmoidoscopy, barium enema, or testing the stool for blood. Forty percent of cancers are too high up in the colon to be reached by the sigmoidoscope. Colonoscopy is performed every 10 years. Virtual colonoscopy with an abdominal CT scan is never correct. It is always the wrong answer.

CLINICAL TIP
The primary care provider needs to be the "quarterback," making sure the specialists are in synch rather than direct prescribing for the patient.

CLINICAL AND EXAM TIP
Bloody stool should always raise a suspicion of colon cancer, especially in smokers and those with a family history of colon cancer.

H. CHOLECYSTITIS

Cholecystitis is the inflammation of the gallbladder. This can come from an outlet obstruction (cholelithiasis or gallstones) or an infection of the gallbladder.

Presentation

The patient usually presents with epigastric or right upper quadrant (RUQ) pain radiating to the back or right shoulder. Pain can radiate from the diaphragm to the shoulder because of the phrenic nerve. Nausea, vomiting, and fever may also present.

Diagnosis

RUQ pain, RUQ tenderness, and fever are fairly specific for cholecystitis. The presence of gallstones on ultrasound or CT scan helps confirm the diagnosis. The hepatobiliary (HIDA) scan is a functional nuclear scan that detects cholecystitis. You should normally be able to visualize the gallbladder with nuclear isotope. An abnormal scan is one in which there is no visualization of the gallbladder.

Treatment

Pain medication, usually a narcotic, is used to control pain. Anti-emetics are used for vomiting. If the gallbladder shows significant signs of infection or a large number of stones, surgical resection of the gallbladder (cholesystectomy) is usually completed. Antibiotics are used for severe acute cases in which the patient is hospitalized.

CLINICAL TIP
Murphy's sign is an abrupt cessation of inspiration from pain when pressure is applied to the RUQ.

I. APPENDICITIS

Appendicitis is the inflammation of the appendix, located in the right lower quadrant (RLQ) of the abdomen. Careful diagnosis of appendicitis must be accomplished: if the appendix bursts, peritonitis (inflammation of the peritoneum) and sepsis may occur.

Presentation

The patient presents with epigastric pain that quickly becomes greatest in the RLQ. Fever, nausea, vomiting, and diarrhea may also occur. Pain and tenderness are greatest at McBurney's point: the point between the right hip and the umbilicus. Signs of appendicitis are given in Table 7-12.

Diagnosis

The white blood count will be elevated. A CT scan with contrast is the best tool to illuminate the appendix. A CT scan that visualizes the appendix has an extremely good negative predictive value. CT scans are 97-98% sensitive.

Treatment

Surgical resection of the inflamed appendix with concurrent antibiotics is the treatment of choice. All patients with an inflamed appendix should be sent to the hospital as the inflammation represents an "acute abdomen." An acute abdomen is an abdominal complaint that will likely require surgical intervention. The following is an equation illustrating the diagnosis of appendicitis:

$$RLQ\ pain + RLQ\ tenderness + Fever + Leukocytosis = Appendicitis$$

TABLE 7-12	Signs of Appendicitis
Dunphy's sign: pain with coughing	
Psoas sign: pain with movement of the leg	

J. DIABETIC GASTROPARESIS

Gastroparesis is a weakness or paralysis of the stomach. The stomach is a muscle. Gastroparesis causes decreased digestion and delayed gastric emptying. Gastroparesis is usually the result of damage to the sensory afferents of the vagus nerve from diabetes. If the stomach can't sense the stretch when food enters it, then motion will not occur.

Presentation

Patients present with nausea, vomiting, and abdominal pain. They may also report early satiety, which means feeling full quickly. Vomitus will likely contain undigested food. Poor appetite, GERD, and bloating may also occur.

This process is related to diabetes in the same manner that peripheral nerve pain occurs with diabetes. Over time, uncontrolled glucose causes nerve damage. No stretch in the stomach is sensed, and therefore there is no appropriate movement.

Diagnosis

Usually no test is needed because gastroparesis is expected in long-term diabetics. When the diagnosis is equivocal, a nuclear gastric emptying study can be done. This involves the patient eating barium-soaked bread and then undergoing imaging to see how long it takes for the bread to empty the stomach.

Treatment

Metoclopromide (Reglan) or erythromycin is given to increase gastric motility. Patients are advised to eat small meals frequently.

K. CELIAC DISEASE: GLUTEN-SENSITIVE ENTEROPATHY

Celiac disease is an autoimmune disorder characterized by chronic abdominal pain, diarrhea, anemia, and fatigue. Weight loss is prominent due to fat malabsorption. Stool is reported as especially foul smelling because of rotting fat in the rectum. In pediatrics, celiac disease can lead to failure to thrive.

The anemia and fatigue associated with celiac disease come from the inability of the intestines to absorb iron, B12, and folate. Celiac disease is also associated with other autoimmune conditions such as diabetes mellitus type 1, hypothyroidism, and Addison's disease.

CLINICAL TIP
Celiac disease is gluten intolerance.

Presentation

Celiac disease is usually diagnosed in childhood. However, in some cases, it can develop in later life. The patient will usually report diarrhea and abdominal cramping. Severe cases have bleeding from vitamin K malabsorption and visual disturbance from vitamin A malabsorption.

Diagnosis

Look for anemia that can be microcytic from iron deficiency or macrocytic from B12 or folate deficiency. Severe cases will have hypocalcemia from vitamin D malabsorption. The prothrombin time is elevated from vitamin K malabsorption. All fat-soluble vitamins, A, D, E, and K, are malabsorbed. Blood tests are presented in Table 7-13.

Referral to gastroenterology and an endoscopy will solidify the diagnosis. Small-bowel biopsy looking for flattening of villi is the most accurate test.

TABLE 7-13	Blood Tests for Celiac Disease
Immunoglobulin A (IgA) anti-tissue transglutaminase (anti-TTG) antibodies	
Anti-gliadin and anti-endomyseal antibodies	

TREATMENT

The treatment for celiac disease is complete avoidance of gluten-containing products. Antispasmodics and antidiarrheals can be used in the short term to alleviate symptoms. Beer, vodka, and whiskey are all wheat derivatives and must be avoided. Wine is okay to drink.

L. ACHALASIA

Achalasia is a dysfunction of the musculature in the distal esophagus. This leads to difficulty with swallowing. There is an inadequacy of relaxation of the lower esophageal sphincter. Achalasia is the opposite of reflux. In reflux, the lower esophageal sphincter is loose and open. In achalasia the sphincter is too tight.

Presentation

Patients present with dysphagia to both solid foods and liquids. The condition gets progressively worse.

Diagnosis

Diagnosis is made with barium swallow studies or EGD. The single most accurate test is the esophageal manometry study.

TREATMENT

The best therapy is either pneumatic dilation with a balloon or surgical myotomy to cut the muscle of the lower esophageal sphincter open. Nifedipine (a calcium channel blocker) can be used to help with relaxing the muscle. Patients should be advised to thoroughly chew their food, to take small bites when they eat, and to sleep elevated. The gastroenterologist should be involved with these patients.

8
Pulmonary

PNEUMONIA

Case 1

A 67-year-old female presents to the nurse practitioner with a history of three days of cough, low-grade fever, fatigue, and congestion. The patient has no past medical history. Her vitals are as follows:

- Blood pressure (BP): 135/89 mm Hg
- Heart rate: 78 beats per minute
- Respiratory rate (RR): 16 breaths per minute
- Temperature: 100.2°F
- Pulse oximetry: 98%

    A chest X-ray shows a left lower lobe infiltrate.

What treatment is appropriate for the patient at this time?

A. Admission for intravenous (IV) antibiotics

B. Azithromycin (Zithromax)

C. Levofloxacin (Levaquin)

D. Amoxicillin/clavulanic acid (Augmentin)

Discussion

The correct answer is B. Macrolides are the primary outpatient treatment of community-acquired pneumonia (CAP). This patient is over the age of 65 but has normal pulse oximetry and a normal respiratory rate. Outpatient treatment should be initiated because the patient is not hypotensive, hypoxic, or confused. If the patient does not improve, becomes hypoxic, develops respiratory distress, or becomes confused, admission for IV antibiotics may be necessary. You do not need to routinely use a fluoroquinolone unless the patient has recently been treated and thus may have more resistant organisms. Table 8-1 lists the sources of pneumonia.

A common source of bacterial pneumonia is *Streptococcus pneumoniae*, which is gram positive. *Haemophilus influenzae* is a gram-negative coccobacillus.

Physical Exam

With pneumonia, there is a possibility of wheezing, crackles, or decreased breath sounds in the affected lobe. The unaffected parts will be normal. Tactile fremitus and whispered pectoriloquy will be increased.

EXAM TIP
Pneumonia = an infection of the lung tissue
Bronchitis = an inflammation of the airways

CLINICAL TIP
Bacterial infections are usually more severe than *mycoplasma*, chlamydia, or viral infections.

TABLE 8-1	Sources of Pneumonia
TYPE OF PNEUMONIA	SOURCE
Lobar (bacterial)	*Streptococcus pneumoniae, Hemophilus*
Bilateral interstitial	*Mycoplasma*, chlamydia, viral
Recent viral syndrome	*Staphylococcus, Pneumococcus*
Hospital acquired	*Pseudomonas*, gram-negative bacilli

Diagnostic Tests

Diagnostic tests for pneumonia are listed in Table 8-2. The best initial test for pneumonia is a chest X-ray.

Treatment

Treatment depends on the patient's comorbidities and the possible cause of the bacteria (ie, type of bacteria). Table 8-3 lists the treatment options for various types of pneumonia.

A tool called the CURB-65, also called the CURB criteria, is often used to predict mortality in community-acquired pneumonia. It assesses the severity of the patient's pneumonia. The name is an acronym for the risk factors measured. Each risk factor scores 1 point, for a maximum score of 5. A score of 2 or more indicates that hospitalization is necessary. Table 8-4 lists the CURB-65 criteria.

Hospital-acquired pneumonia (HAP) will present similarly to community-acquired pneumonia. Table 8-5 lists the guidelines for a diagnosis of HAP.

Treatment for HAP involves a multifactorial approach. Hospital-based bacteria such as *Pseudomonas* are the culprit. Levaquin and other quinolone antibiotics such as moxifloxacin are common in the treatment of HAP. Typically, multiple antibiotics are given intravenously.

TABLE 8-2	Diagnostic Tests for Pneumonia
TEST	REASON
Sputum culture	To identify the specific bacteria and which antibiotics they are sensitive to; that is, to determine which antibiotics will work and which will not
Chest X-ray	Will show infiltration and affected lobes
Complete blood count (CBC)	Will demonstrate white blood cell (WBC) elevation or leukocytosis
Oximeter/arterial blood gas (ABG)	Will show hypoxia, which is a critical criterion for admission

CLINICAL TIP

A comorbidity is another chronic medical problem the patient is experiencing; for example, chronic obstructive pulmonary disease (COPD), coronary artery disease (CAD), diabetes mellitus (DM), liver or renal failure, or alcoholism.

TABLE 8-3	Treatment Options for Pneumonia
TYPE OF PNEUMONIA	TREAMENT
CAP with no comorbidities	Azithromycin
CAP with comorbidities	Levofloxacin, moxifloxacin, amoxicillin/clavulanate potassium
Atypical pneumonia	Azithromycin, clarithromycin
Inpatient therapy	Ceftriaxone and azithromycin

TABLE 8-4	CURB-65 Criteria
Confusion of new onset	
Urea (> 7 mmol/L)	
Respiratory rate > 30 breaths per minute	
Blood pressure < 90 mm Hg systolic or < 60 mm Hg diastolic	
Age > 65	

TABLE 8-5	Hospital-Acquired Pneumonia Diagnosis Guidelines
Hospitalized within 48 hours of onset of symptoms	
Living in nursing home or assisted-living facility	

TABLE 8-6	Medications for Bronchitis	
CLASS		NAME
Mucolytic		Guaifenesin (Mucinex, Robitussin)
Antitussive		Dextromethorphan

CLINICAL TIP
Hypoxia and hypotension are more important than diagnostic tests. If you hear crackles, pneumonia is likely.

EXAM TIP
- Know the difference between bacterial and atypical pneumonia:
  - Atypical pneumonia usually presents as less severe than bacterial pneumonia. Atypical pneumonia is known as "walking pneumonia."
- Azithromycin (Zithromax) is the first line of antibiotics for both bacterial and atypical pneumonia.

BRONCHITIS

Bronchitis is an inflammation of the bronchioles. Inflammation occurs secondary to bacteria, viruses, chemicals, or cigarette smoking. The usual presentation for bronchitis is a persistent non-productive cough, chest congestion, congested breath sounds, and chest tightness.

Treatment

Treatment for bronchitis is symptomatic: mucolytics, antitussive therapy, analgesics, and/or decongestants may be used. Table 8-6 lists some options.

The nurse practitioner must always keep patient safety and comfort in mind. Bronchitis is not associated with morbidity or mortality in its acute phase. If oxygenation is adequate, the patient can be managed in the outpatient setting. Severe disease with discolored sputum and fever is treated as CAP with azithromycin, doxycycline, or sometimes flouroquinolones (eg, levofloxacin, moxifloxacin).

CLINICAL TIP
A vast majority of patients feel the need for antibiotics with bronchitis. This is especially true when the sputum is yellow or green. Patient counseling and education must occur in order not to over-prescribe antibiotics.

PULMONARY EMBOLISM

Case 2

A 25-year-old female presents to the office complaining of shortness of breath and chest pain on deep respiration. The patient recently flew across the country and takes an oral birth control agent.

What is the most appropriate course of action for the nurse practitioner?

A. Start antibiotics

B. Refer to the emergency department (ED)

C. Reassurance

D. Start nebulizer treatment with albuterol

EXAM TIP
Bronchitis is not associated with fever or adventitious breath sounds. If the patient is experiencing either, he or she likely does not have bronchitis.

Discussion

The correct answer is B. There is no indication that there is a bacterial infection, and the patient has obvious risk factors for a pulmonary embolism. She does not have wheezing, which would require albuterol. Reassurance is not appropriate as this patient has risk factors (recent travel, oral birth control agent) and a history compatible with pulmonary emboli. The history you should look for in suspecting an embolus is the sudden onset of shortness of breath with clear lungs.

A pulmonary embolism (PE) begins as a blood clot (thrombus), which is formed and then floats through the blood stream (becoming an embolus), finally becoming lodged in the pulmonary vasculature. This causes a section of the lungs to not receive blood and prevents the gas exchange process.

Presentation

A patient with a PE presents with pleuritic chest pain, shortness of breath, and tachycardia. Hemoptysis (bloody sputum), fever, and crepitations on lung auscultation may be present. Jugular vein distention can be seen on physical exam. The history is very important for this diagnosis. The most important risk factors are prolonged immobility, surgery, trauma, cancer, and especially recent joint replacement.

Deep vein thrombosis (DVT) occurs when a blood clot is formed in one of the body's deep veins; the clot may break loose and travel to the lungs, causing a PE. Patients on oral birth control agents or other hormone-based therapies are also at risk for a PE. PEs and DVT are similar in terms of risks and treatments.

Diagnostic Tests

The best initial tests for a PE are a chest X-ray, electrocardiogram (EKG or ECG), and arterial blood gas (ABG). It is critical to do these tests quickly in any patient with sudden-onset shortness of breath. Initial tests for a PE include the following:

- **D-dimer:** D-dimer is a nonspecific blood test for the presence of a clot. D-dimer is used in low-risk patients to exclude the presence of a PE or DVT. A positive test will not conclusively establish the presence of a clot, or which type of clot if one is present, but a negative D-dimer will exclude the presence of a clot.
- **ABG:** In a patient with a PE, an ABG will demonstrate respiratory alkalosis (an elevation of the blood pH) and a low partial pressure of carbon dioxide (Pco_2). A DVT alone will not alter the ABG.
- **EKG:** The EKG may show tachycardia. An EKG should also be completed to rule out cardiac pathology for dyspnea, another possible symptom of a PE. For example, you need to exclude myocardial ischemia as a cause of dyspnea. When there is an abnormality from PE, the most common are nonspecific abnormalities of the ST and T waves.
- **Chest X-ray:** Most often the chest X-ray in PE patients is normal. It is performed to exclude other reasons for the patient to be short of breath, such as pneumonia or pneumothorax. When there is an abnormality, the most common is atelectasis.
- **Computerized tomography (CT) angiography:** CT angiography of the chest with IV contrast is the most accurate test used to diagnose a PE. This test is important enough that it should be performed even in pregnant patients. Since IV contrast must be given, it is important to evaluate the patient's renal function. Those with borderline renal function need hydration prior to the use of contrast. More severe renal injury means you should consider lower extremity Doppler and/or Ventilation/Perfusion scanning instead to diagnose PE.

Treatment

Anticoagulation is the treatment for a PE. This can be completed in a number of ways. Most commonly in the hospitalized patient with adequate renal function, enoxaparin (Lovenox) is given subcutaneously every 12 hours. Severe renal impairment is a contraindication to the use of enoxaparin.

Oral warfarin (Coumadin) is an anticoagulant that has been around for over 100 years. Patients taking this medication in the hospital must have their international normalized ratio (INR) checked daily via bloodwork. Patients taking oral warfarin on an outpatient basis must have their INR checked weekly. The INR target is between 2 and 3. Oral warfarin should be started while the patient is on heparin.

Rivaroxaban, apixaban, edoxaban, dabigatran are new oral anticoagulants (NOACs) with the following characteristics:

- INR monitoring not needed
- Efficacy equal to or better than warfarin
- Central nervous system (CNS) bleeding as an adverse effect is less frequent with NOACs than with warfarin

Evaluation of Hypercoagulable States (Thrombophilia)

- Protein C, protein S, and factor V Leiden should *not* be performed in the presence of an acute clot. Protein C and S levels are falsely abnormal in the presence of a clot. None of these abnormalities changes either the intensity or the duration of anticoagulation.
- The two forms of thrombophilia most likely to recur are antithrombin deficiency and antiphospholipid syndrome.
- Hematology referral is important.
- Prevention of future clots is important.
- Women on oral birth control medications must be advised to stop such treatment and change their form of birth control, as hormonal agents may cause future clots.

For outpatient tests, ask yourself, "What would I do if the test were positive?" (meaning the patient has a PE). Usually the patient will require inpatient care for a few days. It makes things easier for both the patient and yourself to have the CT performed if the patient is an ED patient.

If the patient has a PE and cannot undergo anticoagulation because of bleeding, placement of an inferior vena cava (IVC) filter should be implanted.

EXAM TIP

If a patient presents with tachycardia, dyspnea, and chest pain, a PE must be ruled out.

CLINICAL TIP

If a PE is suspected, the patient should undergo a STAT chest X-ray and EKG. Next, CT should be performed, or the patient should be sent to the ED.

COUGH

Case 3

A 38-year-old female presents to the office with complaint of a cough lasting 1 month. The cough is worst in the morning, decreasing in severity as the day goes on. The patient has a new dog at home. The patient's vitals are as follows:

- BP: 120/80 mm Hg
- HR: 82 beats per minute
- RR: 16 breaths per minute
- Pulse oximetry: 98%

What is the most likely diagnosis?

A. Pneumonia
B. Allergic rhinitis
C. Upper respiratory tract infection (URI)
D. Sinusitis

Discussion

The correct answer is B. New triggers are a common source of allergies. There is nothing in the history to indicate a bacterial or viral source of infection. Allergies tend to be worse in the morning and improve as the day goes on.

Case 4

A 40-year-old male presents to the office with complaint of a cough lasting for months. He denies any associated symptoms, including fever, postnasal drip, and smoking. The patient works as a chef and states that he likes spicy foods. The patient is diagnosed with gastroesophageal reflux disease (GERD).

What is the proper first-line medication?

A. Famotidine (Pepcid)

B. Pantoprozole

C. Carafate

D. Aluminum hydroxide/magnesium hydroxide/simethicone (Maalox)

Discussion

The correct answer is A. Histamine H2 antagonists (H2 blockers) such as famotidine are first-line therapy for GERD. H2 blockers will control 70% of disease. If they do not work, use a PPI such as omeprazole. All PPIs are equal in efficacy.

Cases 3 and 4 illustrate very different causes of cough. The variety of potential causes of cough must always be present in the mind of the nurse practitioner. Just because a symptom does not have an obvious relation to another system does not mean that it cannot affect another system. Allergies, infection, GERD, and malignancy must always be kept in mind for the differential diagnosis of cough.

Definition

- Cough is a very common presentation to primary care as there are many possible causes for cough.
- Coughing is a normal mechanism for clearing foreign molecules from the upper or lower airway and prevents the body from aspirating potentially harmful substances.
- Common causes of cough include diseases such as chronic obstructive pulmonary disease (COPD), asthma, allergies, postnasal drip, and GERD.
- In recurrent cases in smokers, exclude lung cancer with a chest CT. Even asymptomatic long-term smokers should undergo a chest CT at age 55. This is done annually until age 80.

Presentation

Cough can be acute or chronic. Attention should be paid to whether mucous is being produced and/or expectorated, as well as the color, consistency, and any other characteristics of mucous if present. Causes of cough are listed in Table 8-7.

Diagnostic Tests

- There is no one specific test to diagnose cough.
- Diagnostic tests depend on the presentation of the cough, including its duration, history, and a myriad of other factors.
- A step-wise approach is taken to diagnosis.
- Simple exams, such as a physical, paying special attention to the pharynx, nares, and lungs, are important first steps in the diagnosis of cough.
- A chest X-ray, followed up with other imaging such as CT or magnetic resonance imaging (MRI), can be done.

TABLE 8-7	Causes of Cough
Allergic	
Infectious: bacterial, viral, or parasitic	
Environmental: smoking, cleaning products	
GERD	
Malignancy	
Other: psychogenic, cardiac	

TABLE 8-8	Potential Medications for Cough
CLASS	NAME
Nasal steroid	Mometasone, fluticasone
Nasal anti-allergy	Olopatadine, azelastine
Combination spray	Fluticasone/azelastine
Oral anti-allergy	Loratidine, cetirizine, fexofenadine, levocetirizine
Decongestant	Pseudoephedrine (Sudafed), oxymetazoline (Afrin)
Combination medication	Brompheniramine/dextromethorphan/pseudoephedrine (Bromfed DM)

- Further evaluation by a pulmonologist with pulmonary function tests and direct bronchoscopy can be utilized if necessary.

Treatment

- Treatment depends directly on the cause of the cough.
- Pulmonary causes for cough can be addressed with medications similar to those used for asthma.
- Allergic coughs can be treated with topical steroids such as mometasone or oral anti-allergy medications.
- Cardiac coughs need to be evaluated for type of cardiac condition (eg, congestive heart failure). Cardiac cough involves fluid building up in the lungs and stretching the vessels, which causes the patient cough.

Potential medications for cough are given in Table 8-8.

Referral

- Cough is a primary care condition.
- The initial workup can be done in the primary care setting as can the initial treatment attempts.
- If there is concern or a lack of resolution, arrange a specialist consultation.
- It is important to ensure that there are no underlying and potentially lethal conditions.

CHRONIC OBSTRUCTIVE PULMONARY DISEASE

Case 5

A 70-year-old male presents to the office with persistent cough, dyspnea, and an inability to walk more than 1 city block without stopping to catch his breath. The patient smoked 1 pack of cigarettes per day from age 15 until about 2 years ago. The patient completed an in-office spirometry and has provisionally been diagnosed with chronic obstructive pulmonary disease (COPD).

Which spirometry measurement is most important in the diagnosis of this condition?

A. Forced expiratory volume (FEV1)

B. Total lung volume

C. Residual volume

D. Anatomic dead space

Discussion

The correct answer is A. FEV1 demonstrates the forced expiratory volume in 1 second. This is important for the diagnosis and management of chronic lung pathology. A normal person should be able to exhale at least 80% of the lungs' air in 1 second. In COPD, individuals lose the ability to exhale. That is why this COPD is called an obstructive disease. Although total lung capacity and residual volume increase in COPD, you cannot easily measure them. Anatomic dead space will be normal in a patient with COPD. Anatomic dead space is made up of the bronchi, bronchioles, and trachea.

Diagnostic Tests

- Pulmonary function tests (PFTs) or spirometry will measure the FEV1/FVC ratio.
  - Above 80% is considered satisfactory.
  - Below 80% is considered abnormal and may indicate pathology such as COPD.
- A chest X-ray will demonstrate changes such as decreased compliance or hyperinflation.

Treatment

- Behavior modification is a key first step. If the patient is a smoker, he or she must quit. If the patient lives with a smoker, the smoker must refrain from smoking in the presence of the patient.
- Patients must be educated on the proper use of medication. Patients must be made aware of the differences between short-acting medications for acute attacks and maintenance medications. It is important that patients understand that maintenance medications will not work in acute circumstances.

Medication

- For mild, intermittent symptoms, the best initial therapy is either an inhaled short-acting beta agonist (SABA), such as albuterol, or an antimuscarinic agent, such as tiotropium or ipratropium.
- If neither a SABA nor an antimuscarinic agent effectively controls symptoms, a long-acting inhaled steroid should be added.
- If symptoms are still not controlled following the addition of a long-acting inhaled steroid, a long-acting beta agonist, such as salmeterol, should be added.
  - Long-acting steroids and long-acting beta agonists can be used in combination. Such combinations include mometasone/formoterol (Dulera), budesonide/formoterol (Symbicort), and fluticasone/salmeterol (Advair).
- Home oxygen is used when a patient's sustained oxygen saturation is less than 88% or partial pressure of oxygen (Po_2) is less than 55 mm Hg.

Table 8-9 lists the indications and major side effects of several COPD medications.

CLINICAL TIP

Home oxygen is used when oxygen saturation is less than 90% or PO_2 is less than 60 mm Hg.

TABLE 8-9	Indications and Major Side Effects of COPD Medications	
MEDICATION	INDICATION	MAJOR SIDE EFFECT
Albuterol	Ease dyspnea by relaxing the bronchioles	Tachycardia
Ipratropium	Ease dyspnea by relaxing the bronchioles	Exacerbation of symptoms
Oral steroid (Last resort in outpatient setting)	Decrease airway inflammation	Long-term use associated with bone demineralization
Combination steroid/beta agonist	Decrease airway restriction and inflammation	Exacerbation of symptoms

Referral

- When the patient remains symptomatic despite treatment, referral to pulmonology is warranted.
- If acute exacerbation is suspected as demonstrated by an acute drop in oxygen saturation or dyspnea, an emergency referral is indicated.

ASTHMA

Asthma is a reversible reactive airway disease that causes bronchospasms. Asthma differs from COPD in that it is reversible. Asthma may be idiopathic or have a definitive cause. Table 8-10 lists the causes of asthma.

Presentation

Asthma usually presents with wheezing, shortness of breath, cough, and chest tightness. Increased sputum production and fever may also be present.

Tests

- Peak flow is the best test to determine minute changes in control of asthma symptoms.
- Chest X-rays are usually normal in patients with asthma. There are no specific chest X-ray findings in asthma.
- PFTs will show restriction with small lung volumes, but the FEV1/FVC ratio will be normal. However, note that in asthma, FEV1 will be especially low.

Treatment

A stepwise technique is used in the treatment of asthma:

1. Start with a short-acting beta agonist such as albuterol. Levalbuterol is not superior to albuterol.
2. Add a low-dose inhaled corticosteroid such as beclomethasone, budesonide, flunisolide, fluticasone, mometasone, or triamcinolone.
   - Mast cell stabilizers, such as cromolyn and nedocromil, can also be used. Leukotriene modifiers, such as montelukast, can be used if inhaled steroids cannot.
3. Add a long-acting beta agonist (eg, salmeterol, formoterol) in combination with an inhaled corticosteroid.
   - Long-acting beta agonists are contraindicated in asthma as a solo treatment, as their use in monotherapy may lead to higher asthma-related morbidity and mortality.
4. Maximize the dose of all medications. Add theophylline if maximal inhaled short- and long-acting inhaled steroid and beta agonist treatment continues to be ineffective.
5. Add an oral steroid.

Referral

- When the patient's asthma is not controlled, exacerbations and asthma-related problems require a pulmonology or ED referral.

TABLE 8-10	Causes of Asthma
Infection	
Climate	
Medication side effects	
Tobacco	
GERD	

EXAM TIP
Anticholinergic medications such as ipratropium bromide work well in COPD.

CLINICAL TIP
Patient distress and lack of lung sounds may be signs of severe asthma. Emergency intervention is required.

CLINICAL TIP
There is a link between asthma and eczema.

CLINICAL TIP
Medications for asthma and COPD are very similar in approach and usage.

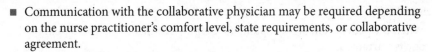

■ Communication with the collaborative physician may be required depending on the nurse practitioner's comfort level, state requirements, or collaborative agreement.

Asthma Exacerbation

■ The basics are key: remember the ABCs.

■ Ensure adequate oxygenation.

■ Oral or parenteral steroids may be indicated.

■ Emergency systems such as 911 may be required.

■ Epinephrine is not better than inhaled beta agonists for acute exacerbations of asthma.

■ The acute rescue medications include the following:
- Inhaled albuterol
- Inhaled ipratropium
- IV or oral steroids
- Magnesium has a modest effect

■ Diminished breath sounds are more ominous than wheezing.

■ Finding the source of the exacerbation is not as important as ensuring the patient is adequately oxygenating.

■ Medications that are *not* effective for acute rescue include the following:
- Montelukast, zafirlukast
- Theophylline
- Cromolyn, nedocromil
- Salmeterol

CLINICAL TIP
- Influenza and pneumococcal vaccines are beneficial in asthma patients.
- Do not use long-acting beta agonists as monotherapy.

TUBERCULOSIS

■ Tuberculosis (TB) is transmitted via respiratory droplets.

■ TB typically affects the lungs but can be found in other sites such as the kidneys.

■ TB tends to be worse for patients with compromised immune systems, such as those with human immunodeficiency virus (HIV), cancer, or diabetes, and those who use steroids.

■ The single most important risk factor for TB is immigration from an endemic country.

■ If TB spreads throughout the body, it is commonly referred to as "military tuberculosis" or "disseminated tuberculosis."

Presentation

■ Fever

■ Bloody, brown, or rust-colored productive cough

■ Weight loss

Organism

■ *Mycobacterium tuberculosis*

Acute Diagnosis

■ **Chest X-ray**: A chest X-ray will show apical infiltrates.

■ **Sputum stain:** An acid-fast stain and culture of the sputum is indispensable in diagnosing TB.
- Do not confuse the procedure for the acute diagnosis of TB with the procedure for the screening of asymptomatic persons with previous exposure. Screening is done via a purified protein derivative (PPD) intradermal skin test or an interferon gamma release assay (IGRA) of the blood.

- **Sputum sensitivity testing**: The sputum stain and culture for acid-fast bacilli allows for sputum sensitivity testing, which is critical prior to beginning treatment.

Treatment

- Acute TB is treated with a combination of isoniazid, rifampin, and pyrazinamide for the first 2 months of therapy.
- After 2 months of treatment, when the organism is sensitive to all medications, a combination of just isoniazid and rifampin is used for a further 4 months.
- The standard of care is to treat for 6 months total.
- The Centers for Disease Control and Prevention (CDC) guidelines advise isoniazid plus vitamin B6 for 9 months.
- Special attention must be given to patients with hepatic compromise. Stop isoniazid when aminotransferase (AST) is 3-5 times the *upper* limit of normal. Once a PPD is positive, do not repeat it, as it will always be positive in subsequent tests.

Screening for Tuberculosis in Asymptomatic Persons

Screening Tests

- A PPD intradermal skin test or IGRA of the blood is the first-line screening procedure for asymptomatic persons. Both the PPD and IGRA are used *only* for screening asymptomatic persons. Neither test is used to establish a diagnosis in an acutely symptomatic person.
- PPD intradermal skin test results will appear as follows:
  - > 5mm for HIV-positive patients, positive close-contact patients, steroid users, and those with a positive chest X-ray
  - > 10mm for immunocompromised patients and healthcare providers
  - < 15mm for general population

Referral

- All PPD-positive patients should be referred to an infectious disease specialist for consultation.

CLINICAL TIP
Previous Bacillus Calmette–Guérin (BCG) vaccination has no impact on treatment recommendations. Forget about BCG. If a patient has received the BCG vaccine and has a reactivity greater than10 mm, he or she will need isoniazid for 9 months.

EXAM TIP
The size of a positive PPD differs based on patient population.

OBSTRUCTIVE SLEEP APNEA

- Obstructive sleep apnea (OSA) is an obstruction of the glottis that occurs while the patient is sleeping.
- OSA is caused by the tongue.
- Patient anatomy plays a role in OSA.

Presentation

- OSA is usually found in overweight or obese patients.
- Snoring is common.
- Patients often complain of fatigue, daytime somnolence, poor sleep patterns, and waking feeling unrested.
- Sometimes it is the spouse of the patient who first notices the patient's snoring.
- Comorbid hypertension and erectile dysfunction may be present, although for unknown reasons.

Diagnostic Tests

- A sleep study is the definitive test for OSA.
- In a sleep study, the patient undergoes electroencephalogram (EEG), electrocardiogram (EKG or ECG), and respiratory pattern monitoring in a controlled setting.

Treatment

- Improve sleep hygiene: Patients are advised not to nap, use their bed only for sleeping, and to get an appropriate amount of sleep each night.
- A bilevel positive airway pressure (BiPAP) or continuous positive airway pressure (CPAP) machine may be used while sleeping.
  - These machines force air into the patient's airway.
  - There are two levels of airway pressure provided by these machines: the BiPAP device gives greater airway support during inhalation than CPAP and is therefore used by patients with more severe OSA.
- Surgery may be performed to open the patient's airway.
- Weight loss is also important in the treatment of OSA.

Referral

Patients with OSA can be referred to pulmonology; ear, nose, and throat (ENT); or dentistry as indicated for treatment:

- Pulmonologists are able to order BiPAP and CPAP machines.
- ENT specialists are used in cases requiring surgical remodeling of the palate.
- Dentists can help with issues caused by the anatomy of the jaw by creating a dental appliance to be inserted at bedtime.

CLINICAL TIP
- Look for complaints of snoring, fatigue, and poor sleep.
- Some recent studies have linked OSA to pathology such as stroke.

CYSTIC FIBROSIS

- Cystic fibrosis (CF) is the most common lethal autosomal-recessive condition in Caucasians.
- CF affects the exchange of sodium and chloride.
- The effects of CF can be seen in the lungs, gastrointestinal and genitourinary tracts.

Presentation

- In childhood, CF may present initially as failure to thrive.
- Patients may experience recurrent upper or lower respiratory tract infections.
- Various vague gastrointestinal complaints, vitamin deficiencies, and/or genitourinary tract abnormalities might be noted.
- Dyspnea, wheezing, cough and large amounts of mucous, may be found on exam.

Cause

- CF is an autosomal-recessive disease.

Diagnostic Tests

- A genetic analysis and CF-specific bloodwork are used to diagnosis CF.
- Tests of the pulmonary system, such as a chest X-ray, PFTs, or ABG, will demonstrate the efficacy of the patient's ventilation and perfusion.

Treatment

- Exacerbations should be treated with bronchodilators such as albuterol.
- Chest physical therapy may be beneficial.
- Pancreatic enzymes should be given to help with vitamin absorption.
- The only definitive treatment for CF is lung transplantation.

CLINICAL TIP
CF can affect fertility, digestion, and many other functions of the body.

Referral

- Referral to pulmonology should be made upon diagnosis.
- Geneticists and other specialists can be consulted as needed.

INFLUENZA

Case 6
A 20-year-old male presents with sudden onset of cough, sneezing, nausea, chills, and fever with a maximum temperature of 38.8°C. The patient states that he is in nursing school and just finished a pediatric rotation.

What is the most likely diagnosis?
A. URI
B. Influenza
C. Sinusitis
D. Viral syndrome

Discussion
The correct answer is B. The sudden onset of symptoms with fever is characteristic of flu, and being around children increases the risk of being exposed.

Symptoms
- Symptoms of flu include coryza (URI-like symptoms such as cough, sneezing, rhinitis, and congestion).
- Viral URIs account for approximately 70-80% of all URIs.

Presentation
- Influenza is an infection of the respiratory and gastrointestinal tracts brought on by an influenza virus. The influenza viruses are classified by their serotype.
- Flu is characterized by a sudden onset of fever, chills, and headache, accompanied by myalgias, fatigue, nausea, vomiting, diarrhea, and abdominal pain or cramping. Coryza may also be present.
- The specific type of influenza virus (whether A, B, or another virus) does not affect presentation or treatment.
  - Treatment is with oseltamivir or zanamivir no matter what organism is responsible.

Diagnostic Tests
- Viral testing can be done for qualitative purposes. A simple nasal swab can be obtained in the office that allows for a diagnosis of influenza type A or B.
- Further cultures or polymerase chain reaction (PCR) can be performed to more specifically identify the virus type.

Treatment
- An antiviral therapy, such as oseltamivir or zanamivir, may be used.
- Antiviral medications must be institute within 48 hours following the onset of symptoms in order to be effective.
- Other types of medication are geared at symptom control.
- Antipyretics are employed to increase patient comfort.

Referral
- Influenza is a primary care condition.
- When the patient becomes hemodynamically unstable, hospitalization should be considered.
- Careful consideration should be given to the very young, the very old, and patients with comorbidities.

CLINICAL TIP
- Oseltamivir must be taken with food.
- Side effects of oseltamivir include nausea, diarrhea, and gastrointestinal upset.
- Oseltamivir works primarily to shorten the duration and lessen the severity of symptoms.

EXAM TIP
- Sudden onset is the key to diagnosing influenza.

9
Hematology and Oncology

The primary care nurse practitioner's scope of practice does not include the diagnosis or treatment of cancers; however, the nurse practitioner must be able to identify danger signs, refer appropriately, and perform proper cancer screenings.

A. BREAST CANCER

Risk Factors
- Family history
- Presence of BRCA1 or BRCA2 gene
- Age at menarche
- Age at menopause
- Obesity
- Smoking
- Alcohol use

Breast Cancer Screening
- Breast cancer screening starts at age 50 unless there is a family history, in which case screening starts 10 years prior to the age of the youngest breast cancer case in the family.
- For those with multiple first-degree relatives (eg, mother, sister) with breast cancer, tamoxifen can be used to decrease the risk of breast cancer by 50%. Tamoxifen would be given entirely as preventive therapy in this case.

Signs and Symptoms
- Lump in breast
- Enlarged axillary lymph nodes
- Nipple discharge
- Change in texture or size of breast

Diagnosis
- Diagnosis is made via biopsy, mammogram, magnetic resonance imaging (MRI) scan, and/or ultrasound of the breasts.
- A sentinel lymph node is the first lymph node to which cancer cells are most likely to spread from a primary tumor. It is the key to determining if the entire axilla needs to be dissected to assess the lymph nodes for the presence of cancer.

CLINICAL TIP

A lump is present in only 20% of breast cancer cases.

CLINICAL TIP

You can never go wrong by sending a patient for a mammogram or ultrasound when there is a breast complaint.

CLINICAL TIP

The missed diagnosis of breast cancer is one of the most common medical liability cases.

■ In a sentinel lymph node biopsy (SLNB), a dye is injected into the area to see which node picks it up first. If that first, or "sentinel," lymph node does *not* show cancer, the axilla does *not* need to be dissected.

Treatment

■ Breast cancer patients should be under the care of a hematologist/oncologist.

■ Chemotherapy and radiation are used for the treatment of breast cancer.

■ A modified radical mastectomy (the surgical removal of breast tissue and surrounding tissue) may be performed.

■ The combination of lumpectomy and radiation are just as effective as modified radical mastectomy in most patients.

■ Patients with positive estrogen or progesterone receptors on biopsy require treatment with tamoxifen, raloxifene, or an aromatase inhibitor.

■ Patients who express extra receptors require treatment with anti-HER2/neu antibody therapy (trastuzumab).

■ Patients with a lesion greater than 1 cm in diameter or with metastases to the lymph nodes require chemotherapy.

■ Support should be given to the patient and his or her family. Counseling and psychology referrals should be made as indicated.

B. PROSTATE CANCER

■ The overall cause of prostate cancer is unclear.

Risk Factors

■ Age

■ Family history

■ Race (more prevalent in the African American population, but a higher death rate in the Caucasian population)

■ Smoking

Screening

■ There is no definitive screening test for prostate cancer.

■ A prostate-specific antigen (PSA) blood test is of no clear benefit in screening but remains the primary screening tool for prostate cancer.

■ A digital rectal exam (DRE) (manual palpation of the prostate gland) is unable to find cancer at a stage at which meaningful intervention can occur.

Signs and Symptoms

■ Nocturia

■ Hematuria

■ Dysuria

■ Rectal discomfort

■ Change in urine stream

■ Painful erection or ejaculation

Diagnosis

■ A normal PSA level is < 4 ng/mL. Levels above 4 ng/dL indicate the possibility of prostate cancer.

■ It is important to monitor for PSA level (the number) as well as PSA velocity (the change in number over time).

■ On DRE, a normal prostate gland should be small, rubbery, and nontender.

■ Biopsy is required for accurate diagnosis.

■ MRI and ultrasound can be used for further evaluation.

Treatment

- Prostate cancer patients should be under the care of a urologist and hematologist/oncologist.
- Upon diagnosis of prostate cancer, PSA can be measured at intervals to assess the rate of growth of the cancer. Rising PSA levels indicate the need for biopsy. This is *not* the same as using PSA for screening.
- Treatment options include radiation and surgical removal of the prostate.
- Surgical removal of the prostate is superior to radiation in younger patients with a high Gleason score (which demonstrates aggressive pathology).

CLINICAL TIP
15% of all males will have some stage of prostate cancer by age 80.

C. LUNG CANCER

Risk Factors

- Smoking
- Second-hand smoke
- Genetic predisposition
- Environmental factors (eg, asbestos exposure)

Signs and Symptoms

- Persistent cough, sometimes bloody or blood-tinged
- Wheezing or dyspnea
- Weight loss
- Fatigue
- Pain (related to mass)

Diagnosis

- Lung cancer patients will usually present with a long history of cough.
- Lung cancer initially presents with symptoms similar to pneumonia that do not improve with antibiotics.
- On plain X-ray exam, a nodule or mass may be present. Lymph node involvement is also often present.
- Lesion biopsy is needed for final diagnosis and staging.

CLINICAL TIP
A computerized tomography (CT) scan or MRI can be used to further visualize the nodule, mass, and/or lymph nodes.

Treatment

- Lung cancer patients should be under the care of a hematologist/oncologist and pulmonologist.
- Treatment consists of a combination of chemotherapy, radiation, and surgical removal of the mass or affected lung.
- The key factor guiding therapy is the possibility of surgically removing the cancer, as only surgery can cure lung cancer (Table 9-1).
- Chemotherapy and radiation reduce the growth rate of lung cancer, but they do not eradicate the cancer.
- Ensure that a smoking cessation program is in place.

CLINICAL TIP
- In the case of any persistent cough, send the patient for chest X-ray.
- Initiate a smoking cessation program.

EXAM TIP
Keep lung cancer in mind for questions about persistent cough.

TABLE 9-1	When a Lung Tumor Cannot be Resected
Heart, vena cava, or aorta involvement	
Malignant pleural effusion	
Bilateral disease	
Esophageal involvement	

D. COLON CANCER

Risk Factors

- Smoking
- Alcohol use
- Family history
- Low-fiber, high-fat diet
- History of inflammatory bowel disease (IBD)

Screening

- Colon cancer screening begins at age 50.
- The best screening test is colonoscopy.
- Sigmoidoscopy misses the 40% of cancers that are beyond the reach of the sigmoidoscope.
- Fecal occult blood testing and barium enema still require colonoscopy.
- The fecal occult blood test requires the collection of three stool samples.

Signs and Symptoms

- Blood in the stool
- Weight loss
- Fatigue
- Nausea, vomiting
- Constipation

Diagnosis

- Diagnosis is made via biopsy completed by a gastroenterologist during a colonoscopy.

Treatment

- Treatment options include chemotherapy, radiation, and the removal of the mass or affected portion of the colon.

CLINICAL TIP

Even if the patient has an identifiable cause for blood in the stool (eg, hemorrhoid), a gastroenterology (GI) evaluation should be considered to rule out further pathology.

EXAM TIP

Safety is key. For questions concerning blood in the stool, the answer is likely the one that provides the safest option for the patient.

E. LYMPHOMA AND LEUKEMIA

- Lymphoma is cancer of the lymph system.
- Leukemia is cancer of the white blood cells produced by the bone marrow.

Risk Factors

- History of immunosuppression (eg, HIV/AIDS)
- Epstein-Barr virus
- Smoking
- Radiation exposure

Signs and Symptoms

- Fever
- Weight loss
- Fatigue
- Painful, swollen lymph nodes
- Anemia
- Frequent infections (as a result of a weakened immune system)

Diagnosis

- The diagnosis will be definitive from a biopsy of the bone marrow or lymph node.

- In a lymph node biopsy, the entire node should be removed. This is called an excisional biopsy.
  - Needle biopsy is used in the case of infections (eg, bacterial infection, tuberculosis).

Treatment

- Lymphoma and leukemia patients should be under the care of a hematologist.
- Treatment options include radiation, chemotherapy, and bone marrow transplant.
- Bone marrow transplantation allows for a much higher dose of chemotherapy.
- Patients with non-Hodgkin's lymphoma are tested for CD20 antigen. If CD20 is present, rituximab is added to the treatment regimen to increase the clearance of the lymphoma.
- In lymphoma and leukemia, infection prevention is extremely important as these are disorders of the white blood cells.

Adverse Effects of Chemotherapy

It is important to be aware of the long-term adverse effects of chemotherapy:

- Vincristine/vinblastine: peripheral neuropathy
- Bleomycin: lung fibrosis
- Doxorubicin: cardiac toxicity
- Cyclophosphamide: hemorrhagic cystitis

F. MULTIPLE MYELOMA

- Multiple myeloma is the cancer of plasma cells.

Signs and Symptoms

- Bone pain/fracture (occurs in 70% of patients)
- Fever (as a result of dysfunctional white cells)
- Fatigue (as a result of anemia)
- Frequent infections as a result of dysfunctional plasma cells

Lab Abnormalities

- Elevated calcium
- Renal failure
- Anemia
- Bone lesions; lytic lesions found on X-ray

Diagnosis

- X-ray of affected bone(s)
- Serum protein electrophoresis (SPEP): monoclonal elevation of a single type of immunoglobulin G (IgG)
- Urine electrophoresis: Bence Jones protein

Treatment

- Melphalan with prednisone
- Combination chemotherapy
- Lenalidomide or thalidomide
- Under age 70, autologous bone marrow transplantation with stem cell support
  - An autologous transplant is a type of transplant that uses the patient's own stem cells, which means that there will be no rejection or graft-versus-host disease.
- In multiple myeloma, infection prevention is extremely important as it is a disorder of the white blood cells.

G. ANEMIA

- "Anemia" is a blanket term describing a decrease in red blood cells.
- Red blood cell volume is measured via hemoglobin and hematocrit.
- Iron, vitamin B12, and folate deficiencies and thalassemia are common causes of anemia.

Signs and Symptoms

- Fatigue, weakness, malaise, tachycardia, palpations, dyspnea, and shortness of breath on exertion are common symptoms of anemia.
- Vague, nonspecific symptoms are also possible.
- In severe cases, patients may experience altered mental status.
- All symptoms result from a deficiency of hemoglobin in the blood; hemoglobin is needed to deliver oxygen to the body's tissues.
- It is not possible to determine the cause of anemia from the presenting symptoms.

Diagnosis

- Checking the conjunctiva or mucous membranes for pallor may aid in the diagnosis of anemia.
- Once anemia is noted, mean corpuscular volume (MCV) is the next step taken to determine the source of the anemia (Tables 9-2 and 9-3).

TABLE 9-2	Mean Corpuscular Volume
MEAN CORPUSCULAR VOLUME	TYPE OF ANEMIA
< 80 fL	Microcytic anemia
> 100 fL	Macrocytic anemia
80-100 fL	Normocytic anemia

TABLE 9-3	Types of Anemia	
TYPE OF ANEMIA	COMMON CAUSES	TREATMENT
Microcytic anemia	Iron deficiency Thalassemia Sideroblastic anemia (abnormal production of red cells) Lead poisoning	Iron deficiency: iron replacement Other causes: treatment of underlying condition
Macrocytic anemia	Vitamin B12 deficiency Folate deficiency Bone marrow cancer	Vitamin B12 deficiency: Vitamin B12 replacement Folate deficiency: folate replacement Other causes: treatment of underlying condition
Normocytic anemia	Anemia of chronic disease (often occurs in dialysis patients) Sickle cell anemia Blood loss, hemolysis	Treatment of the underlying condition

TABLE 9-4	Drugs to Avoid in G6PD Deficiency
CLASS	EXAMPLES
Sulfa medications	Bactrim
Antimalarial medications	Chloroquine, primaquine
Analgesics	Acetylsalicylic acid (aspirin)
Antibiotics	Isoniazid, nitrofurantoin, dapsone

Referral

- Referral to hematology may be considered for resistant or refractory anemia.
- Patients with anemia related to thalassemia, sickle cell, or glucose-6-phosphate dehydrogenase (G6PD) deficiency should be evaluated by hematology.
- Patients with hemoglobin < 8 g/dL should be evaluated in the emergency department (ED) as they will likely require a blood transfusion.

H. G6PD DEFICIENCY

- Glucose-6-phosphate dehydrogenase (G6PD) deficiency is an X-linked recessive genetic condition.
- Because G6PD deficiency is an X-linked recessive genetic condition. Generally only, males are affected.
- G6PD deficiency results in hemolysis following exposure to certain foods (eg, beans and legumes), infections, or drugs, especially sulfa drugs (Table 9-4).
- Hemolysis is the rupture of red blood cells.
- Hemolysis results in jaundice, which is the yellowing of the skin and eyes.

Diagnosis

- Patients will likely present with jaundice, bleeding, or hemolysis.
- Blood tests should be performed to check for hemolysis.
- A Coombs test will detect autoimmune disease from the presence of antibodies against red blood cells.
- A haptoglobin test will show abnormally low levels of haptoglobin.
  - Haptoglobin transports newly released hemoglobin from dead red blood cells to the liver to be recycled.
- A lactate dehydrogenase (LDH) test will show increased LDH levels, indicating increased red blood cell destruction.

Treatment

- Patients with G6PD deficiency should be under the care of a hematologist.
- There is no specific therapy for G6PD deficiency except for avoidance of oxidative stresses.
- Blood transfusions are performed in severe cases.
- Steroids may be used as G6PD is an autoimmune disease.
- In cases of sideroblastic anemia, patients should avoid drinking alcohol. Some may respond to vitamin B6 (pyridoxine).

I. COAGULOPATHY

When a patient presents with bleeding, the two most important questions to ask in your assessment are as follows:

- Is the bleeding related to a platelet disorder (low platelet count or platelet dysfunction) or clotting factor disorder (Table 9-5)?
- How much blood has been lost?

CLINICAL TIP

Determine the type of bleeding *before* initiating blood tests.

CLINICAL TIP

Bleeding of the gastrointestinal (GI) tract or central nervous system (CNS) can occur as a result of either platelet or clotting factor disorders.

TABLE 9-5	Platelet Disorder versus Clotting Factor Bleeding	
PLATELET DISORDER		**CLOTTING FACTOR DISORDER**
Superficial bleeding		Deep bleeding
• Epistaxis		• Hemarthrosis (joint)
• Petechiae, purpura		• Hematoma (muscle)
• Gingiva (gums)		
• Menstrual		

IA. Von Willebrand Disease

- Von Willebrand disease involves platelet-type bleeding with a normal platelet count.
- Von Willebrand disease results either from a deficiency of Von Willebrand factor (VWF) or from a defect in its function.
- Von Willebrand factor (VWF) is synonymous with factor VIII antigen.
- The condition worsens with the use of acetylsalicylic acid (aspirin).
- Von Willebrand disease is lifelong and recurrent.
- There is often a family history.

Diagnosis

- The patient's VWF level should be measured, and a ristocetin cofactor assay (a test of the function of the VWF) should be performed.
- 50% of patients will have an elevated activated partial thromboplastin time (aPTT) because the defective VWF destabilizes the factor VIII coagulant (hemophilia A factor).
- A test of bleeding time is rarely done any more. In this test, the patient is made to bleed and the time it takes to stop bleeding is measured.

Treatment

- Initial therapy is with desmopressin.
- If there is no response to desmopressin, the patient will undergo factor VIII replacement. Recombinant VWF can also be used.

IB. Immune (Idiopathic) Thrombocytopenic Purpura

- Immune (idiopathic) thrombocytopenic purpura (ITP) is a profoundly low platelet count.
- ITP is characterized by bleeding occurring when the platelet count is less than 10 000-20 000 per microliter.
- The spleen is of normal size.
- The white blood cell (WBC) count and differential will be normal.

Diagnosis

- ITP is a diagnosis of exclusion; there is no definitive test to diagnose ITP.
- Bone marrow biopsy is done to exclude a production defect when the diagnosis is not clear from the history. Look for increased megakaryocytes to diagnose ITP.

Treatment

- When a patient presents with isolated thrombocytopenia and a normal-sized spleen, do not delay starting therapy in order to complete tests.
- Prednisone is the best initial therapy.
- If recurrences are frequent after stopping steroids, a splenectomy should be performed.
- Life-threatening bleeding requires intravenous immunoglobulin (IVIG) therapy.
- Following splenectomy, recurrences are managed with romiplostim or eltrombopag.

CLINICAL TIP
Factor VIII contains VWF.

CLINICAL TIP
Don't delay treatment waiting for bone marrow.

CLINICAL TIP
Antiplatelet antibodies do *not* help in ITP.

CLINICAL TIP
IVIG is used for intracranial and major GI bleeding.

IC. Warfarin Overdose Vitamin K Deficiency, and Liver Disease

- Warfarin overdose, vitamin K deficiency, and liver disease present identically with an elevation of prothrombin time (PT), aPTT, and international normalized ratio (INR).

Treatment

- Fresh frozen plasma (FFP) is the fastest way to reverse the effect of warfarin and stop bleeding. Prothrombin complex concentrate (PCC) replaces all vitamin K dependent factors, 2, 7, 9, 10 and quickly reverses warfarin toxicity.
- If there is bleeding with any of these disorders, give FFP immediately.
- FFP lasts for only for a few hours, up to a day at most.
- Patients with vitamin K deficiency require vitamin K replacement.
- In cases of warfarin overdose, the decision to use vitamin K replacement is based on whether the patient will be continuing warfarin therapy later on but at a lower intensity. If the patient will *not* be continuing warfarin therapy, vitamin K replacement can be given in addition to FFP.

ID. Disseminated Intravascular Coagulopathy

- Disseminated intravascular coagulopathy (DIC) presents with bleeding as a result of both platelet loss and clotting factor deficiency. Because of this, bloodwork will show an elevation in both PT and aPTT and a low platelet count.
- If the platelet count is greater than 50 000 per microliter, platelets do not need to be given.
- DIC does not appear by itself but as a complicating factor from an underlying condition. Look for major conditions or diseases, such as the following:
  - Sepsis
  - Cancer
  - Leukemia
  - Amniotic fluid embolus

Diagnosis

- Elevated PT, aPTT, and INR
- Decreased platelet count
- Elevated D-dimer and fibrin split products (FSP)
- Decreased fibrinogen
- Signs of hemolysis are common: increased LDH, reticulocytes, and indirect bilirubin
- Fragmented cells (schistocytes and helmet cells) on smear

Treatment

- Treatment is with FFP.
- Platelets are given when the platelet count is less than 50 000 per microliter and the patient is bleeding.
- Heparin is *not* useful.

IE. Heparin-Induced Thrombocytopenia

- Heparin-induced thrombocytopenia (HIT) is a greater than 50% reduction in platelets with the use of any amount of heparin.
- Usually occurs a few days after the use of heparin
- With enoxaparin (a low-molecular-weight heparin [LMWH]), there is less risk of HIT, but not zero risk.
- Do *not* wait for antiplatelet factor 4 antibodies or the serotonin release assay to stop heparin treatment.
- If full-dose anticoagulation is needed (eg, in the case of pulmonary embolism [PE]), fondaparinux is used.

CLINICAL TIP

FFP is the fastest way to reverse warfarin overdose if bleeding is present.

CLINICAL TIP
Patients who have experienced HIT after receiving IV heparin cannot simply be switched to an LMWH.

CLINICAL TIP
Even small doses of heparin, such as those used in a flush or deep vein thrombosis (DVT) prophylaxis, can cause HIT.

CLINICAL TIP
A mixing study corrects aPTT to normal after a 50:50 mix or patient plasma with normal plasma with those with a clotting factor deficiency. Those with a clotting factor inhibitor would still have an elevated aPTT after the 50:50 mix with normal plasma.

- Fondaparinux is an Xa inhibitor that is easier to use than the direct thrombin inhibitor argatroban.
- HIT can cause *both* venous and arterial thrombosis.
There will still be a chance or HIT with the switch to LMW heparin.

IF. Clotting Factor Deficiencies: Hemophilia

- In hemophilia, joint bleeding is delayed 1-2 days following the trauma.
- The primary hemostatic plug consists of platelets, which will dissolve if fibrin is not produced to solidify the plug.
- aPPT will be increased aPTT; PT will be normal.
- aPTT can be corrected to normal upon mixing with normal plasma.
- Mild disease is treated with desmopressin.
- Severe disease is treated with factor VIII or IX replacement as needed.

IG. Hypercoaguable States: Thrombophilia

- DVT and PE are common diagnoses.
- DVT is treated almost exclusively on an outpatient patient basis via subcutaneous injection of an LMWH followed by warfarin for 6 months.
- The INR target for both DVT and PE is 2-3.
- Evaluation for thrombophilia is not necessary during an acute episode of thrombosis.
- Factor V Leiden mutation is the most common inherited cause of thrombophilia.
- Regardless of the cause of the thrombophilia (ie, factor V Leiden mutation, protein C or S deficiency, antithrombin deficiency), the intensity and duration of coagulation are the same.
- The only thrombophilic state that may alter management is antiphospholipid syndrome (APS).
  - APS is sometimes called anticardiolipin antibody syndrome or lupus anticoagulant syndrome.
  - APS may require lifelong treatment even when only one clot is present.

J. SICKLE CELL ANEMIA

- Sickle cell anemia is a form of anemia in which the red blood cells are abnormally shaped in the form of a sickle.
- Sickle cell anemia causes severe pain.
- Severe infections may occur because the spleen becomes damaged by the sickle-shaped cells.
- Sickle crisis occurs when blood flow is blocked by sickled cells that have become stuck in blood vessels, thus reducing blood flow to organs and tissues (Table 9-6).

Diagnosis

- The first test in sickle cell anemia diagnosis is a smear; sickle-shaped cells will be seen.
- Hemoglobin electrophoresis is the most accurate test for any hemoglobinopathy such as sickle cell disease. You should expect to see:
  - Elevated LDH and indirect bilirubin levels
  - Elevated reticulocyte count
  - Decreased haptoglobin level

Indicators of Severe Sickle Crisis

- Low reticulocyte count = aplastic crisis
- Fever or WBC count higher than usual = dangerous infection

CLINICAL TIP
Sickle cell anemia predominately affects individuals of African descent.

TABLE 9-6	Types of Sickle Crisis
TYPE OF SICKLE CRISIS	**DESCRIPTION**
Vaso-occlusive	Causes extreme pain Treatment includes hydration and analgesia Transfusion is sometimes required Crises in end-organ areas (eg, penis, lungs) are medical emergencies
Acute chest syndrome	Diagnosis requires two of the following: chest pain, fever, pulmonary infiltrate, respiratory symptoms, hypoxemia Accounts for 25% of deaths in patients with sickle cell anemia
Aplastic crisis	Worsening of baseline anemia Pallor, fatigue, tachycardia, and weakness are commonly seen Parvovirus B19 can be a cause Blood transfusion may be required in cases of significant anemia

CLINICAL TIP
A sickle crisis is often precipitated by infection, dehydration, or acidosis.

CLINICAL TIP
Sickle cell anemia is part of the mandatory blood panel completed at birth.

Referral

- Following diagnosis, patients should be referred to hematology for further management.

Treatment

- Hydration, oxygen, and pain medications are the mainstays of treatment.
- In cases of fever or high WBC count, antibiotics are given (eg, ceftriaxone, levofloxacin).
- Hydroxyurea is given to prevent sickle crises. Raise the dose of hydroxyurea until there is >15% hemoglobin F.
- Vaccinations are very important in the pediatric population.
- All individuals with sickle cell anemia should receive folic acid.
- Hemoglobin monitoring for patients with sickle cell anemia is well within the scope of the primary nurse practitioner's role.

K. THALASSEMIA

- Thalassemia is a blood disorder involving abnormally formed hemoglobin cells.
- As a result of the abnormally formed hemoglobin cells, oxygen transport is decreased and hemolysis occurs.
- Individuals with thalassemia trait carry the genetic trait for thalassemia but rarely experience any health problems as result except perhaps for a mild anemia called microcytic anemia.

Diagnosis

- Thalassemia is diagnosed via hemoglobin electrophoresis.
- In beta thalassemia, the following will be noted:
  - Decreased hemoglobin A (HbA)
  - Increased HbF
  - Increased HbA_2
- In alpha thalassemia, the following will be noted:
  - Normal electrophoresis
  - Three genes deleted: HbH (beta 4 tetrads)
  - Genetic studies required for definitive diagnosis
- There is no treatment for thalassemia trait.

10
Nephrology: Sodium Disorders

A. DIABETES INSIPIDUS AND SYNDROME OF INAPPROPRIATE ANTIDIURETIC HORMONE SECRETION

- Diabetes insipidus (DI) and syndrome of inappropriate antidiuretic hormone (SIADH) secretion have similar presentations because they are both sodium disorders.
- DI occurs when there is a decrease in the amount of antidiuretic hormone (ADH) secreted or when there is a problem with the ADH receptors at the collecting duct of the kidney:
  - Decreased ADH production is called central diabetes insipidus (CDI).
  - The inactivity of V2 receptors in the kidney is called nephrogenic diabetes insipidus (NDI). NDI is caused by either hypercalcemia or/and hypokalemia.

AA. Diabetes Insipidus

- Both CDI and NDI present with increased urine production and thirst because the body is unable to retain the water it needs.
- Both CDI and NDI present with hypernatremia.
- Urine sodium and urine osmolarity will be low. The rate at which sodium rises is associated with the severity of symptoms: the faster sodium rises, the worse the symptoms.
- Symptoms include confusion, disorientation, and malaise.
- Seizures and coma can be later signs and symptoms in severe cases.

Treatment

- Any patient demonstrating symptoms of a sodium disorder should be sent to the emergency department (ED).
- Symptomatic hypernatremia requires hydration.
- CDI requires ADH replacement therapy with vasopressin.
- Nephrogenic DI generally resolves with the correction of calcium and potassium.
- All DI patients should be referred to nephrology.

AB. Syndrome of Inappropriate Antidiuretic Hormone

- SIADH is hyponatremia from abnormal free water retention without edema.
- The presentation of SIADH is similar to DI: confusion, malaise, disorientation, and, in severe cases, seizures and coma.

- As in DI, the rate at which sodium drops is associated with the severity of symptoms: rapid drop in sodium results in worse symptoms.

Etiology

It is *critical* to determine the cause of SIADH in the patient because effective treatment relies on correcting the underlying cause:

- Central nervous system (CNS): Many possible sources, including stroke, tumor, head trauma, seizure, and pain
- Lungs: Many possible sources, including infection, emboli, cancer, and atelectasis
- Medications
- Cancer

Diagnostic Diagnostic Tests

- Serum sodium will be low (hyponatremia).
- Serum osmolarity will be low.
- Urine sodium will be abnormally high: > 20 mEq/L/24 h.
- Urine osmolarity will be abnormally high: a value > 100 mOsm/kg is high if the patient is hyponatremic.

Treatment

- Mild SIADH will present with low sodium but no symptoms. Fluid restriction will correct the sodium level.
- Severe SIADH will present with confusion and altered mental status. Treatment is with 3% hypertonic saline and an ADH antagonist such as conivaptan or tolvaptan.

B. DIABETIC NEPHROPATHY

- Diabetic nephropathy is a progressive kidney disease that occurs in individuals with diabetes.
- The disease results from damage to capillaries in the kidneys' glomeruli, which results in protein loss.
- The severity of diabetic nephropathy ranges from asymptomatic proteinuria to end-stage renal failure.

Diagnostic Tests

- The first diagnostic test that should be performed is a urinalysis (UA). The UA will detect protein only when the protein level goes above the equivalent of 300 mg/24 h.
- Normal protein levels in the urine are < 50 mg/24 h.
- A urine protein level between 50 mg/24 h and 300 mg/24 h is called microalbuminuria. Microalbuminuria cannot be detected on the urine dipstick.

Treatment

- Strict glucose control in diabetes is imperative.
- Medications such as angiotensin-converting enzyme inhibitors (ACEIs) or angiotensin receptor blockers (ARBs) should be used in patients with diabetes to prevent the onset of nephropathy characterized by a rising creatinine level.

CLINICAL TIP
Patients with diabetes should be screened annually for proteinuria.

EXAM TIP
- Patients with type 2 diabetes should be screened for proteinuria upon diagnosis.
- Patients with type 1 diabetes should be screened 5 years after diagnosis.

C. PYELONEPHRITIS

- Pyelonephritis is an infection of the kidney and upper urinary tract.
- It is usually caused by an obstructing kidney stone or untreated cystitis.
- The presenting symptoms are flank pain, fever, abdominal pain, nausea, and vomiting.

- Hydronephrosis, the swelling of the kidney as a result of urine build-up, may accompany pyelonephritis.
- Fluid in the ureter may also accompany pyelonephritis.

Diagnostic Tests

- The best initial diagnostic test is a UA looking for white blood cells (WBCs).
- Although a urine culture will tell you the specific organism and sensitivities, it will not tell you if a kidney infection is present.
- Imaging such as a computerized tomography (CT) scan or ultrasound will demonstrate inflammation of the kidney. Imaging is performed to identify correctable causes of pyelonephritis.

Treatment

- Third-generation cephalosporins, such as ceftriaxone, or quinolone antibiotics are usually given.

CLINICAL TIPS

If patients can tolerate an oral diet and oral medications, they can usually be treated as outpatients.

D. RENAL FAILURE

- There are two categories of renal failure: acute and chronic.
- Acute kidney injury is defined by a sudden decrease in creatinine clearance, which leads to an elevation in blood urea nitrogen (BUN) and creatinine.
- There are 3 types of acute kidney injury:
  - **Prerenal azotemia:** decreased perfusion (eg, hypotension, hypovolemia, shock)
  - **Postrenal azotemia:** obstruction (eg, kidney stone, prostate disease)
  - **Intrinsic renal disease:** kidney death (eg, due to gentamicin or other drug toxicity)
- Patients rarely present for "kidney failure," but rather with symptoms such as fatigue, nausea, pruritus, weakness, or other vague complaints. Acute tubular necrosis (ATN) is one form of acute renal failure. It is almost always from a combination of decreased renal perfusion and nephrotoxic agents.
- The nurse practitioner should use clinical clues, such as blood pressure, heart rate, and how the patient presents before deciding if the patient should be referred to the ED or to outpatient nephrology.

Stages of Chronic Kidney Disease

- The stages of chronic kidney disease are presented in Table 10-1.

TABLE 10-1	Stages of Chronic Kidney Disease	
STAGE	GLOMERULAR FILTRATION RATE (GFR) (mL/min/1.73m²)	TREATMENT
CKD 1	90+	Monitor Control comorbid conditions
CKD 2	60-89	Strict dietary and medication compliance
CKD 3	GFR 30-59	Continue strict monitoring Assess for risk of cardiovascular damage
CKD 4	GFR 15-29	Continue all steps of stages 1-3 Assess need for dialysis
CKD 5	GFR < 15	Dialysis

Diagnostic Tests

- Testing BUN and creatinine levels is the first step in assessing the etiology of acute kidney injury.
- Prerenal azotemia is defined by a BUN/creatinine ratio of 20:1. Urine sodium will be low (< 20 mEq/L/24 h), and urine osmolarity will be high (> 500 mOsm/kg).
- When the kidney injury is inside the kidney (intrinsic), the BUN/creatinine ratio will be closer to 10:1. Urine sodium will be higher (> 40 mEq/L/24 h), and urine osmolality will be lower (< 350 mOsm/kg).

Treatment

- Chronic kidney disease is the result of a precipitating cause, such as diabetes or hypertension, and progresses over time.
- Once the kidneys have suffered a degree of death, dialysis is required.
- Dialysis is a process that takes over the role of the kidneys, using either the patient's blood or peritoneum to filter out toxins and excess fluids, tasks the kidneys can no longer perform.
- There is no medication to reverse acute tubular necrosis (ATN).
  - Treatment for ATN consists of stopping exposure to the relevant toxin to prevent further damage.
  - Once injury has occurred, you must wait to see if recovery occurs; in severe cases, assess whether dialysis is needed.
- Correct the underlying cause.
- Hydration is helpful in most cases.

Contrast Agents

- There is no treatment to reverse injury to the kidneys with contrast agents; the only management is to prevent the injury.
- One to two liters of half-normal or normal (isotonic) saline is given in advance of the procedure and again 6 hours after the procedure.
- N-acetylcysteine may help.
- Sodium bicarbonate may help.
- The only true preventive therapy is hydration.
- Hydration is not given to every patient receiving contrast agents. It is given only to those who have underlying renal dysfunction with an elevated creatinine level, such as those with diabetes or hypertension and those who are elderly.

CLINICAL TIP
Once chronic kidney disease is established, the patient should be seen regularly by a nephrologist.

CLINICAL TIP
Loop diuretics (eg, furosemide) are ineffective and potentially dangerous in ATN.

E. RHABDOMYOLYSIS

Case 1

A 30-year-old female patient presents with diffuse muscle pain and cramping. She has been training for an upcoming marathon. She states that she has been drinking water in appropriate amounts to her level of exercise. On microscopic examination, her urine dipstick is positive for blood but negative for red blood cells. Her urine is grossly tea colored.

What is the most likely diagnosis?

A. Urinary tract infection (UTI)

B. Kidney atone

C. Pyelonephritis

D. Rhabdomyolysis

Discussion

The correct answer is D. Rhabdomyolysis is the breakdown of muscle fibers from extreme exercise (among other causes). Blood without red blood cells is a common finding in rhabdomyolysis. Rhabdomyolysis is caused by trauma, poisoning, or injury that increases myoglobin filtering through the kidneys.

Patients with rhabdomyolysis typically present with back pain, diffuse myalgias (muscle pains), and dark-colored urine. The key to diagnosis is a history of muscle injury, seizure, or prolonged immobility.

Diagnostic Tests

- Urinalysis: The urine dipstick will be positive for blood but with no red blood cells present. (The urine dipstick cannot distinguish between hemoglobin, myoglobin, or red blood cells.)
- A urine test for myoglobin and a blood test for creatine kinase (CK) may also be done.
- BUN and creatinine will be elevated.
- Potassium will be elevated, possibly to a fatal level.
- Calcium will be low because damaged muscle binds calcium. (The damaged muscle will also release phosphate.)

Treatment

- Treatment is via hydration with normal saline.
- Bicarbonate and mannitol may also be used. Bicarbonate protects the kidneys and drives potassium into cells.
- The patient must be monitored for acidemia as the kidneys may alter the body's acid-base balance.

Referral

- Patients with rhabdomyolysis should be sent to the ED for intravenous (IV) fluids with a request for a nephrology consultation.

F. NEPHROLITHIASIS

Case 2

A 29-year-old male presents to the primary care nurse practitioner complaining of sudden, severe right flank pain. On exam there is tenderness with palpation to the costovertebral angle (CVA) on the right side. This pain radiates around the right flank toward the groin. The physical exam is otherwise normal. A urine dipstick is completed and is normal except for blood.

What is the most likely diagnosis?

A. UTI
B. Nephrolithiasis (kidney stone)
C. Pyelonephritis
D. Muscle spasm

Discussion

The correct answer is B. Kidney stones present with sudden onset of unilateral flank pain. Blood is commonly present in the urine because of trauma to the urinary tract from the stone. The patient reports no fever or dysuria, which would have indicated pyelonephritis or UTI. Muscle spasm presents with a less focused presentation.

Kidney stones are formations of material, most commonly calcium oxalate, which usually forms in alkaline urine. Patients with nephrolithiasis typically present with severe flank pain and occasionally nausea or vomiting.

CLINICAL TIP
Dark urine with only protein should undergo further workup.

CLINICAL TIP
History is very important in the diagnosis of rhabdomyolysis; patients typically report having recently exercised more than usual or having been recently injured.

EXAM TIP

For questions related to nephrolithiasis diagnosis, X-ray is the most common *wrong* answer. An abdominal X-ray is used only to detect small-bowel obstruction. A CT scan is the most accurate diagnostic test for nephrolithiasis.

CLINICAL TIP

Patients will experience pain only when the stone is in the ureter or urethra.

CLINICAL TIP

If the stone is greater than 5-7 mm in diameter, a urological procedure is typically required to remove the stone. Stones between 5 mm and 20 mm in diameter are treated with shock wave lithotripsy (SWL).

Diagnostic Tests

- CVA pain will be present in most clinical presentations of nephrolithiasis.
- A CT scan or ultrasound will be the next step following physical exam. A CT scan is the most accurate diagnostic test for nephrolithiasis.

Treatment

- A nonsteroidal anti-inflammatory drug (NSAID), commonly ketorolac, will be prescribed for pain and to decrease inflammation.
- Narcotic pain medication for analgesia should be used to keep the patient comfortable.
- Antibiotics are used when infection is present.
- A vasodilating medication, such as tamsulosin or nifedipine, is given to both male and female patients when the diameter of the urethra needs to be increased.
  - 90% of stones smaller than 5 mm in diameter will pass spontaneously.
  - Larger stones (6-7 mm) can pass with the aid of tamsulosin or nifedipine.

11
Endocrinology

A. DIABETES MELLITUS TYPES 1 AND 2

- Diabetes mellitus is a metabolic disease characterized by abnormalities in the regulation of blood glucose, in which the hormone insulin is either not secreted, secreted in too small an amount, or the body's cells are resistant to the hormone.

- Type 1 diabetes occurs when the beta cells of the pancreas do not secrete insulin. This is most commonly the result of an autoimmune process.

- Type 2 diabetes occurs when the pancreas does not produce enough insulin or the body's cells are resistant to insulin.

- There are several types of medications for type 2 diabetes management. The role of each is to lower blood glucose levels; however, the mechanism of action differs greatly among the medications available.

CLINICAL TIP
It is because the body does make some insulin that individuals with type 2 diabetes do not always require insulin therapy.

Diagnosis

- Remember the 3 Ps: polydipsia, polyphagia, and polyuria.
- Also watch for the following signs and symptoms:
  - Unexplained and non-resolving conditions
  - Nausea
  - Vomiting
  - Diarrhea
  - Abdominal pain
  - Paresthesia
  - Recurrent infections (eg, cellulitis)
  - Changes in hair or skin

Diagnostic Tests

- A fasting glucose of > 125 mg/dL or a hemoglobinA1c (HbA1c) of > 6.5% is consistent with a diagnosis of diabetes.
- An HbA1c < 7 on treatment is considered controlled diabetes.
- A single glucose level of > 200 mg/dL in the presence of symptoms also establishes a diagnosis of diabetes.
- Oral glucose tolerance testing is used in pregnant women to test for gestational diabetes.

TABLE 11-1 | Diabetes Medications

CLASS	NAME	MECHANISM OF ACTION
Sulfonylurea	Glimepiride, glipizide, glyburide	Stimulates insulin secretion Increases absorption of insulin Increases gluconeogenesis
Biguanide	Metformin	Decreases hepatic glucose production
Thiazolidinedione	Pioglitazone, rosiglitazone	Decreases insulin resistance Allows for increased glucose absorption
Dipeptidyl peptidase-4 (DPP-4) inhibitor	Alogliptin, linagliptin, saxagliptin, sitagliptin	Slows incretin metabolism Increases insulin synthesis/release Decreases glucagon level
Sodium-glucose cotransporter 2 (SGLT2) inhibitor	Canagliflolzin, dapagliflozin, empagliflozin	Inhibitis SGLT2 Reduces glucose reabsorption Increases urinary glucose excretion
Glucagon-like peptide-1 (GLP-1) analog	Liraglutide Exenatide, Dulaglutide	Activates GLP-1 Increases insulin secretion Decreases glucagon production Delays gastric emptying (producing early satiety)
Meglitinide	Nateglinide, repaglinide	Increases insulin level after eating
Insulin	Regular: insulin regular human (Humulin, Novolin) Short-acting: insulin lispro (Humalog), insulin aspart (NovoLog) Long-acting: neutral protamine Hagedorn (NPH) Combination short- and long-acting (basal): glargine/detemir	Always subcutaneous (regular insulin is the only one that can be administered intravenously) Provide insulin for patients who cannot make their own supply (used in both types 1 and 2) Used in type 2 diabetes when oral therapies fail Regular and short-acting used for short-term coverage (insulin pump, postprandial dosing) Long-acting and combination short- and long-acting prescribed with daily or twice-daily (bid) dosing to maintain steady insulin levels throughout the day

CLINICAL TIP

Diet education is very important for all patients with diabetes.

EXAM TIP

Type 2 diabetes, more often than type 1 diabetes, has a genetic basis.

Treatment

- Type 1 diabetes is always treated with insulin as the patient's pancreas does not produce any insulin.
- Type 2 diabetes is treated with a combination of lifestyle modifications including diet (low starch and sugar intake) and exercise. Medications are usually oral in the beginning, transitioning to injectable as the condition becomes more severe (Table 11-1). Insulins are used once lifestyle modifications are no longer effective.

Referral

- Types 1 and 2 diabetes can be treated by the primary care provider.
- When the patient can no longer be managed by the primary care advanced practice nurse (APN), a referral to endocrinology should be made.

B. THYROID DISORDERS

- The thyroid is an endocrine gland that controls the body's metabolism.
- The thyroid gland is located in the lower anterior neck.
- The anterior pituitary gland is responsible for the secretion and function of the thyroid gland.

TABLE 11-2	Hypothyroidism Signs and Symptoms
Dry, coarse skin and hair	
Fatigue	
Cold intolerance	
Weight gain	
Constipation	
Poor memory	

TABLE 11-3	Hyperthyroidism Signs and Symptoms
Weight loss	
Irritability	
Heat intolerance	
Palpitations	
Tremors	
Anxiety	
Gastrointestinal (GI) disturbances	

- Hypothyroidism occurs when the thyroid is underactive (Table 11-2).
- Hyperthyroidism occurs when the thyroid is overactive (Table 11-3).
  - Graves disease, an autoimmune disorder, is the most common cause of hyperthyroidism.

Treatment

- Treatment for hypothyroidism is hormone replacement therapy. Levothyroxine is most commonly used.
- Treatment for hyperthyroidism is more complex.
  - Grave's disease is treated with beta blockers, which help to prevent the signs and symptoms of hyperthyroidism (ie, tremors, tachycardia, hypertension).
  - Propranolol is a commonly used beta blocker for Grave's disease treatment.
  - Other medications for hyperthyroidism includes propylthiouracil (PTU) and methimazole.
  - PTU is the drug of choice for pregnant women with hyperthyroidism.

CLINICAL TIP
Hyperthyroidism is a very common cause of fatigue, hair loss, and inability to conceive.

EXAM TIP
Thyroxine (T4) is down when thyroid-stimulating hormone (TSH) is up; T4 is up when TSH is down.

C. PHEOCHROMOCYTOMA

- Pheochromocytoma is a tumor of the adrenal gland.
- This tumor secretes large quantities of catecholamines such as epinephrine and norepinephrine.
- The tumor is usually unilateral but can occasionally be bilateral.

Diagnosis

- The patient will likely present with new-onset hypertension, arrhythmia, or other hemodynamic instability.
- During the workup of these symptoms, catecholamine testing is completed.
- Elevated levels of catecholamines in a 24-hour urine test establish the diagnosis of pheochromocytoma.

CLINICAL TIP

Always remember to evaluate the patient for pheochromocytoma during workup for primary hypertension.

EXAM TIP

A 24-hour-urine test is the most sensitive diagnostic tool for pheochromocytoma.

CLINICAL TIP

I once had a patient who presented with persistent vomiting and pneumomediastinum (air in the mediastinum) after vomiting, who ended up with hyponatremia (sodium: 107 mg/dL). He was admitted to the hospital where a serum ACTH was completed, and he was diagnosed by endocrinology with Addison's disease.

CLINICAL TIP

Be on the lookout for increased cortisol and decreased serum ACTH.

Referral

- Referral to an endocrinologist and surgeon will help determine the final diagnosis and appropriate treatment.

Treatment

- Treatment consists of modulating the abnormal hormone levels and surgical removal of the tumor if possible.

D. ADDISON'S DISEASE

- Addison's disease is an autoimmune endocrine disorder in which the adrenal glands hyposecrete steroid hormones such as glucocorticoids and mineralocorticoids.
- The current prevalence of the disease is 100 per 1 million.
- Patients typically present with a sudden onset of nausea, vomiting, and low blood pressure, which may occur following trauma or illness or may be idiopathic.

Diagnostic Tests

- Testing will reveal an elevated serum adrenocorticotropic hormone (ACTH) level with a low cortisol level.
- Low sodium and glucose levels and a high potassium level may also be found.

Referral

- Patients should be referred to endocrinology or admitted to the hospital.

Treatment

- Treatment consists of serum cortisol (intravenous [IV] hydrocortisone) replacement.

E. CUSHING'S SYNDROME

- Cushing's syndrome is a syndrome of increased cortisol in the blood, commonly from ACTH-secreting tumors in the pituitary gland.
- Cushing's syndrome is commonly caused by the prolonged use of steroids.
- Patients typically present with depression, insomnia, obesity, weight gain, change in menstrual cycle (females), change in libido, and/or weakness.

Signs and Symptoms

- Round face
- Stretch marks
- Increased posterior fat pads
- Elevated blood pressure
- Central obesity
- Myalgia
- Muscle weakness

Diagnostic Tests

There are two steps to establishing a diagnosis of hypercortisolism:

1. Establish that cortisol is high but without establishing the source.
2. Locate the source of the high cortisol.

   The tests to establish the presence of hypercortisolism include the following:

- The 24-hour urine cortisol test is the most accurate diagnostic test.
- The 1 mg overnight dexamethasone suppression test measures whether ACTH secretion by the pituitary gland can be suppressed. A normal response is the suppression of morning cortisol.
- Midnight salivary cortisol levels may also be tested. A normal result is low salivary cortisol.

Sources of High Cortisol

- Adrenal source: low ACTH and elevated cortisol
- Pituitary source: high ACTH, which can be suppressed with high-dose dexamethasone
- Ectopic or cancerous source: high ACTCH that *cannot* be suppressed with high-dose dexamethasone

Referral

- Patients should be referred to endocrinology.
- A hematology/oncology consultation may be required if a pituitary tumor is thought to be involved.

12

Genitourinary

URINARY TRACT INFECTIONS

- A urinary tract infection (UTI) is an infection of the lower urinary tract.
- UTIs are commonly caused by bacteria, most often *Escherichia coli* (*E. coli*) (Table 12-1).
- There is a much higher incidence of UTIs in women than men; however, men can also experience UTIs.
- Cystitis is the infection and inflammation of the bladder.
- Pyelonephritis occurs when the infection reaches the kidneys.
- Patients with a UTI usually present with urinary discomfort, frequency, and urgency.
- Occasionally, patients may present with suprapubic pain, nausea, fever, and hematuria (blood in the urine).

CLINICAL TIP
The most common cause of UTIs is the bacterium *E. coli*.

Risk Factors

- Age: The elderly have a higher risk of contracting a UTI.
- Urinary catheters
- Sexual activity in women (high risk)
- Anatomic structural abnormalities

Diagnosis

- Urinary frequency, urgency, and burning sensation are usually enough to establish a diagnosis.
- Leukocytes (white blood cells) and nitrites will be present on urinalysis.

TABLE 12-1	Bacteria that Cause Urinary Tract Infections
Escherichia Coli	
Staphylococcus saprophyticus	
Klebsiella	
Proteus	
Pseudomonas	

- If leukocytes are present in the urine of a symptomatic female, nitrites do not need to be present to establish a diagnosis.
    - Nitrites are a metabolic end product of gram-negative bacteria.
- A urine culture is not necessary in cases of uncomplicated cystitis.

Treatment

- Antibiotics are required to treat UTIs.
- The most commonly used antibiotics are nitrofurantoin and sulfamethoxazole/trimethoprim.
- Nitrofurantoin is the antibiotic given mostly during pregnancy.
- Amoxicillin is given to pediatric patients.
- Quinolones are reserved for cases of recurrent UTI or drug resistance. Quinolones are used sparingly in the treatment of UTIs to avoid increased drug resistance.
- Phenazopyridine, a urinary tract anesthetic, may be given to alleviate discomfort.

Referral

- UTI is a primary care diagnosis that can be accurately diagnosed and treated by the nurse practitioner.
- A referral to urology can be considered after recurrent UTIs.
- Occasionally a urogynecologist is consulted if a fistula between the gastrointestinal (GI) and genitourinary (GU) tracts is suspected.

SEXUALLY TRANSMITTED DISEASES

Gonorrhea

- Gonorrhea is one of the most common sexually transmitted diseases (STDs).
- Gonorrhea is caused by the bacterium *Neisseria gonorrhoeae*.
- In men, symptoms usually present as discharge and a burning sensation on urination.
- Women may be asymptomatic or present with vaginal discharge or pelvic pain.

Diagnosis

- Diagnosis is based on clinical history and polymerase chain reaction (PCR) testing.
- A PCR test is done on urine voided into a cup in men and via a patient self-administered swab in women.

Treatment

- First-line treatment consists of a one-time intramuscular dose of ceftriaxone.

Chlamydia

- Chlamydia is caused by the bacterium *Chlamydia trachomatis*.
- Chlamydia is a common STD worldwide.
- There is a 50% chance that women with chlamydia will be asymptomatic.
- When symptoms do occur in women, dyspareunia (painful sexual intercourse), fever, painful urination, urinary frequency, vaginal bleeding, and a thin, yellowish vaginal discharge are common.
- Men with chlamydia experience symptoms of urethritis (pain on urination). A discharge, usually yellowish in color, may also be present.
- There are various modes of chlamydia transmission (Table 12-2).

Diagnosis

- Diagnosis is based on clinical history and PCR testing.
- As in gonorrhea, a PCR test is done on urine voided into a cup in men and via a patient self-administered swab for women.

CLINICAL TIP
A urine culture and sensitivity analysis will determine the species of the bacterium and the antibiotics susceptible, important to know in cases of recurrent infection.

EXAM TIP
Know the difference between upper (flank pain) and lower (suprapubic pain) UTIs.

CLINICAL TIP
Phenazopyridine is helpful for symptom control. Advise patients that it will turn their urine orange.

CLINICAL TIP
Gonorrhea is becoming more resistant to antibiotics, so treatment must be followed by a repeated PCR test.

CLINICAL TIP
Untreated chlamydia is a leading cause of pelvic inflammatory disease.

TABLE 12-2	Modes of Chlamydia Transmission
Oral sex	
Anal sex	
Vaginal sex	
Maternal to fetal	

Treatment

- Directly observed therapy (DOT) is recommended.
- Treatment is most often with the antibiotic azithromycin, given orally.
- Doxycycline is also used.

Pelvic Inflammatory Disorder

- Pelvic inflammatory disorder (PID) is the inflammation of the uterus, fallopian tubes, and/or ovaries.
- PID is usually the cause of STDs, such as chlamydia and gonorrhea, in women.
- Common symptoms include lower abdominal pain, fever, cervical motion tenderness, vaginal discharge, dyspareunia, or vaginal bleeding.

Treatment

- Outpatient therapy consists of ceftriaxone and doxycycline.
- Inpatient therapy consists of intravenous (IV) cefoxitin or cefotetan and doxycycline.

Trichomoniasis

- Trichomoniasis is a common STD caused by the protozoan parasite *Trichomonas vaginalis*.
- As in chlamydia and gonorrhea, trichomoniasis can be asymptomatic.
- When symptoms do occur, itching or irritation inside the penis or vagina, a burning sensation, erythema, and soreness are common.
- Women may present with dyspareunia.
- Men may present with discharge.
- A white, yellow, clear, or green malodorous discharge may be noted. Both men and women have a discharge.

Treatment

- Metronidazole is the drug of choice for trichomoniasis infections.

Human Immunodeficiency Virus

- Human immunodeficiency virus (HIV) is an STD causing progressive failure of the immune system and, over time, acquired immune deficiency syndrome (AIDS).
- Without treatment, patients die from opportunistic infections that their compromised immune systems cannot protect against.
- CD4 T cells are the most affected by the virus.
- Macrophages and dendritic cells are also affected.
- HIV is often asymptomatic. The first symptoms to appear are generally viral upper-respiratory-like symptoms.
- Do not ask about risk factors; simply test every adult patient.

Treatment

- Medications used in the treatment of HIV are presented in Table 12-3.
- It is valid to treat every patient, even those whose CD4 count is above 500 cells/μL.

CLINICAL TIP

If you treat for gonorrhea, treating for chlamydia is indicated as well.

CLINICAL TIP

Screening exams by a gynecologist or family practice nurse practitioner will often catch gonorrhea or chlamydia in time to prevent PID.

CLINICAL TIP

There is an interaction between metronidazole and alcohol. Patients are advised to avoid alcohol during treatment and for at least 3 days following completion of treatment.

CLINICAL TIP

The U.S. Preventive Services Task Force (USPSTF) recommends screening for HIV during annual exams.

TABLE 12-3 | HIV Medications

CLASS	NAME
Protease inhibitor	Atazanavir, lopinavir/ritonavir, ritonavir
Non-nucleoside reverse transcriptase inhibitor (NNRTI)	Efavirenz, rilpivirine
Integrase inhibitor	Dolutegravir, elvitegravir/cobicistat, raltegravir
Pharmacokinetic enhancer	Ritonavir
Nucleoside/nucleotide reverse transcriptase inhibitors (NRTI)	Abacavir/lamivudine, tenofovir/emtricitabine

CLINICAL TIP
HIV becomes AIDS when the CD4 count falls below 200 cells/µL.

CLINICAL TIP
Combination therapy is critical. Patients with HIV typically require a treatment regimen including at least 3 drugs.

EXAM TIP
HIV is asymptomatic until the CD4 count is significantly below 200-350 cells/µL. Do not wait for this drop in CD4 to initiate treatment.

- The standard of care is to combine two nucleoside reverse transcriptase inhibitors (NRTIs), such as emtricitabine and tenofovir, with an integrase inhibitor, such as dolutegravir, raltegravir, or elvitegravir.
  - Elvitegravir is combined with cobicistat, which inhibits the metabolism of the integrase inhibitor.
- The alternative to a nucleoside foundation is a combination of abacavir and lamivudine with an integrase inhibitor.
  - Abacavir can only be used in patients who do not experience a Stevens-Johnson-type allergic skin reaction, which involves testing for human leukocyte antigen (HLA) B5701. If this mutation is present, do not use abacavir.

Referral

- Once a diagnosis is made, the patient should be referred to an infectious disease specialist.
- The primary care provider should be alert for any signs or symptoms of opportunistic infection.

Pregnancy and HIV

- Don't ask about risk factors; simply test all patients.
- Treat every pregnant patient, no matter how high the CD4 or how low the viral load.

Human Papillomavirus

- Human papillomavirus (HPV) is a viral infection of the genital tract.
- HPV is the most common STD.
- HPV varies in its clinical presentation and significance. Some strains can cause cervical cancer, others cause warts, and still others have no clinical presentation.
- Most strains of HPV are entirely asymptomatic.
- HPV is spread through sexual activity: vaginal, anal, and oral.

Treatment

- Warts can be treated by a dermatologist. Liquid nitrogen, laser, and podophyllin are used to melt the warts, and imiquimod is used as a painless local immunostimulant.

CLINICAL TIP
Vaccination is worthwhile even in individuals who are already sexually active as they may not yet have acquired the potentially carcinogenic strain of the virus.

Prevention

- Prevention against certain strains is possible via the HPV quadrivalent (types 6, 11, 16, and 18) recombinant vaccine, given in a series of 3 doses.
- This vaccine protects against the strains most commonly associated with cervical cancer.

Syphilis

- Syphilis is an STD caused by the spirochete bacterium *Treponema pallidum*.
- There are 4 stages of presentation of syphilis (Table 12-4).

TABLE 12-4	The Four Stages of Syphilis Presentation
STAGE	PRESENTATION
Primary	Painless chancre
Secondary	Diffuse rash on palms of hands and soles of feet
Latent	No symptoms
Tertiary	Neurologic and cardiac symptoms

Diagnostic Tests

- Rapid plasma reagin (RPR) and venereal disease research laboratory (VDRL) are the screening tests for syphilis. They are equivalent in accuracy.
- If the RPR or VDRL test is positive, a confirmatory test is completed: fluorescent treponemal antibody absorption (FTA-ABS).
- For primary syphilis, the most accurate diagnostic test is dark-field examination.
  - RPR and VDRL are only 70-80% sensitive in primary syphilis.
- For neurosyphilis, the most accurate test is cerebrospinal fluid fluorescent treponemal antibody (CSF-FTA). A negative CSF-FTA absolutely excludes neurosyphilis.

Treatment

Primary and Secondary Syphilis

- First-line therapy for primary and secondary syphilis is a single dose of benzathine penicillin (penicillin G), given intramuscularly.
- In cases of penicillin allergy, doxycycline is used.

Tertiary Syphilis

- If the patient has progressed to tertiary syphilis prior to treatment, IV penicillin for a minimum of 10 days is required.
- In the case of penicillin allergy, the patient must be desensitized to penicillin.
- Due to the spirochete nature of the bacterium, a reaction called the Jarisch-Herxheimer reaction occurs shortly after treatment is rendered. This reaction is characterized by headache, myalgia, tachycardia, and fever.

CLINICAL AND EXAM TIP
- Painless genital lesions indicate primary syphilis.
- Painful lesions are herpetic.

Herpes Simplex Virus

- Herpes simplex virus (HSV) is a viral infection caused by the herpes virus.
- HSV can be associated with oral or genital herpes no matter what subtype is involved.
- HSV is transferred through direct contact.
- Once the virus is introduced to the body, there is no cure; the virus may only be suppressed with a reduction in the outward display of lesions.
- HSV lesions are painful and ulcerated.
- There are various types of herpes infection (Table 12-5).

TABLE 12-5	Types of Herpes Infection
Herpes labialis (cold sores)	
Genital herpes (blisters on the genital mucosa; STD)	
Herpes zoster (shingles)	
Herpes keratitis (eye infection; an ophthalmologic emergency)	

Diagnostic Tests

- For genital herpes, the most accurate diagnostic test is PCR. Viral culture is not as sensitive.
- For herpes zoster (shingles) or a reactivation of varicella zoster virus, a swab with PCR is performed. The same is true for herpes simplex. Herpes keratitis is fluorescein staining of the cornea. Keratitis can be confirmed with PCR as well

Treatment

- Treatment is focused on viral suppression via antiviral medications.
- The most commonly used antiviral medications are acyclovir, famciclovir, and valacyclovir.
- The medications used are the same no matter the location of the infection.
- Oral therapy is essential; topical therapy is useless.

CLINICAL AND EXAM TIP

Herpes lesions are painful.

CLINICAL TIP

Some patients may require antifungal medication after receiving antibiotics.

CLINICAL TIP

The most common fungus involved in fungal vaginitis is *Candida albicans* (*C. albicans*).

FUNGAL VAGINITIS

- Fungal vaginitis (yeast infection) is a fungal infection of the vagina.
- Fungal vaginitis may occur as a primary infection or secondary to antibiotic use.
- Patients at high risk for yeast infections are those who are immunocompromised; for example, those with cancer, HIV, or diabetes, and those who have undergone organ transplantation.
- Fungal vaginitis infections present as a white area with surrounding erythema.
- Patients typically describe the affected area as itchy, irritated, sore, or burning.
- A white or gray cottage cheese–like or curd-like discharge may be present.
- Candida infections do not have the "fishy" odor characteristic of bacterial vaginitis caused by *Gardnerella vaginalis*.

Diagnosis

- Diagnosis is made via history and physical exam.
- Swabs of the discharge or tissue can also be acquired for microscopic analysis.
- Using potassium hydroxide (KOH), *C. albicans* can be visualized. KOH melts away the epithelial cells so that only fungal hyphae are visible.

Treatment

- Antifungal treatment can be topical or oral.
- Common topical agents include clotrimazole, nystatin, fluconazole, and ketoconazole.
- A common oral medication is fluconazole.
- Note: Metronidazole is *not* used for fungal vaginitis. Metronidazole is used for bacterial vaginitis.
- Dosing and strength depend on the clinical picture.
  - For example, a healthy female with a yeast infection following antibiotic treatment may require only a single oral dose of fluconazole 150 mg, whereas a patient with HIV or one who has undergone organ transplantation may require 10 days of oral therapy.

EXAM TIP

Remember the characteristic white or gray cottage cheese–like or curd-like discharge.

BACTERIAL VAGINITIS

- Bacterial vaginitis (BV) is an infection of the vaginal mucosa that typically occurs following douching or as a result of having multiple sexual partners (Table 12-6).
- BV is not considered an STD. Rather, it is thought to occur as result of a change in the vaginal flora.
- Patients often present with a sticky, white or off-white discharge accompanied by a "fishy" odor.
- Patients may complain of slight itching or irritation and localized erythema.

CLINICAL TIP

Douching is one of the major causes of BV.

TABLE 12-6	Common Causes of Bacterial Vaginitis
Gardnerella vaginalis	
Mycoplasma hominis	
Ureaplasma urealyticum	

Diagnostic Tests

- Diagnosis is made via whiff test, in which several drops of a KOH solution are added to a sample of vaginal discharge to see whether a strong "fishy" odor is produced.
- The pH of the vaginal mucosa will also be elevated (more alkaline in comparison to its usual acidic level).

Treatment

- Metronidazole or clindamycin are commonly used for treatment.
- These medications can be given orally or intravaginally.

CLINICAL TIP

One-time dosing is no longer recommended for BV.

CLINICAL AND EXAM TIP

A "fishy" odor is characteristic of BV.

13
Men's Health

A. PROSTATE CANCER SCREENING

- Screening via routine prostate-specific antigen (PSA) testing and digital rectal examination (DRE) is not to be done.
  - PSA testing misses many cancers and overdiagnoses prostate cancer.
  - PSA screening has been given a class "D" recommendation from the U.S. Preventive Services Task Force (USPSTF), which means PSA screening is not helpful and possibly harmful.
- The prostate should feel like a pencil eraser.
- If the prostate is warm, tender, or painful, consider infection.
- If the prostate is enlarged but not painful, the patient should be followed up for benign prostatic hyperplasia versus cancer.

Diagnostic Tests

- When the prostate is enlarged, a biopsy should be completed by a urologist to determine a benign versus malignant process.

Referral

- Patients should be referred to urology for any abnormal bloodwork or physical exam findings to rule out and/or catch early prostate cancer.

B. BENIGN PROSTATIC HYPERPLASIA

- Benign prostatic hyperplasia (BPH) is a benign enlargement of the prostate gland.
- BPH can cause nocturia (having to get up at night to urinate), a decrease in urine flow, and urinary discomfort.
- BPH typically presents in middle age.
- Typical complaints include a decreased intensity of urine flow, the inability or difficulty with starting urine flow, or dribbling urine.

Diagnostic Tests

- A physical exam is the first-line method for detecting an enlarged prostate.
- PSA testing is still recommended by the Centers for Disease Control and Prevention (CDC) and the American Cancer Society, but its validity is currently being questioned.

TABLE 13-1	Benign Prostatic Hyperplasia Medications
CLASS	NAME
Alpha blocker	Alfuzosin, doxazosin, silodosin, tamsulosin, terazosin
5-ARI	Dutasteride, finasteride

CLINICAL TIP

Alpha blockers can cause orthostatic hypotension (a drop in blood pressure upon standing.

CLINICAL TIPS

Know the size and texture of a normal versus abnormal prostate gland.

EXAM TIP

Despite the final diagnosis being made by the urologist, the correct exam answer will discuss the nurse practitioner being involved in the patient's assessment. Referral alone will *not* be the correct answer.

CLINICAL TIP

Prostatitis is considered a medical emergency.

CLINICAL TIP

Prostatitis treatment is typically given for 3 weeks.

EXAM TIP

A warm, tender prostate signifies prostatitis; an enlarged, boggy prostate signifies BPH.

■ If any results are abnormal, the patient should be referred to a urologist, who will perform a biopsy on the prostate to check for cancer.

Treatment

■ Treatment consists of alpha blockers (commonly used for initial therapy) and 5-alpha-reductase inhibitors (5-ARIs) (Table 13-1).

Referral

■ If there is anything abnormal on physical exam or PSA test, the patient should be referred to urology.

■ Rapid referral and biopsy are key to early diagnosis and treatment if cancer is present.

C. PROSTATITIS

■ Prostatitis is the inflammation of the prostate gland, usually due to a bacterial infection (Table 13-2).

■ Patients typically present with pain and urinary frequency and urgency.

■ Fever and rectal pain may also be present.

Treatment

■ Intravenous (IV) antibiotics are usually given in the acute setting. IV ceftriaxone or quinolones are most common.

■ The patient is then transitioned to oral therapy for 3 weeks.

■ The medications used for prostatitis are the same as those used in cystitis; however, they are used for longer in prostatitis.

Referral

■ A urology consultation is usually recommended during the acute stage of prostatitis.

■ It is also beneficial for the patient to be followed by urology during the recovery stage in order to prevent recurrence or chronic prostatitis.

TABLE 13-2	Common Bacteria in Prostatitis
Escherichia coli	
Klebsiella	
Proteus	
Pseudomonas	
Enterobacter	
Enterococcus	
Staphylococcus aureus	

D. TESTICULAR TORSION

- Testicular torsion is the twisting of the spermatic cord.
- Testicular torsion is an acutely painful emergent condition.
- If not corrected, the affected testicle will become ischemic and die.
- Patients typically present with a sudden onset of severe unilateral testicular pain and a lack of cremasteric reflex.
  - The cremasteric reflex is the contraction of the scrotum when the inner thigh is stimulated.

Diagnostic Tests

- An emergent ultrasound should be completed. In testicular torsion, this will demonstrate a lack of blood flow to the affected testicle and will show the spermatic cord twisted.
- On physical exam, look for one elevated testicle.

Treatment

- The only treatment for testicular torsion is surgical correction.

Referral

- Patients should promptly be sent to the emergency department (ED) for an immediate urological and surgical evaluation and treatment.

CLINICAL TIP

If testicular torsion is not corrected within 6 hours, the testicle will likely need to be removed.

E. EPIDIDYMITIS

- Epididymitis is an inflammation of the epididymis causing pain. The epididymis is where the sperm mature.
- Epididymitis is most often caused by a bacterial infection (Table 13-3).
- Patients typically present with an acute onset of testicular or scrotal pain.
- Urinary discharge or dysuria may also occur.
- The pain associated with epididymitis differs from the pain associated with testicular torsion. In epididymitis, the cremasteric reflex remains intact, and the pain is relieved upon elevation of the testes.

Diagnostic Tests

- Since epididymitis presents similarly to testicular torsion, an ultrasound is usually warranted to differentiate the two.
- Look for testicular tenderness in epididymitis (versus the one elevated testicle in testicular torsion).

Treatment

- If the patient is sexually active and the cause of the epididymitis is chlamydia or gonorrhea (or both), treatment should be to eradicate the chlamydia or gonorrhea (or both). Treatment consists of ceftriaxone and azithromycin.
- For non-STD-related epididymitis, common UTI antibiotics can be used (eg, ciprofloxacin, trimethoprim/sulfamethoxazole [TMP/SMZ]).

CLINICAL AND EXAM TIP

Patients will present with acute unilateral testicular pain. The cause may be either traumatic or atraumatic.

CLINICAL TIP

Epididymitis differs from testicular torsion. In epididymitis, pain is relieved when the testicles are elevated.

CLINICAL TIP

Epididymitis is commonly caused by gonorrhea and chlamydia. It may also be caused by UTI bacteria such as *E. coli*.

TABLE 13-3	Common Bacteria in Epididymitis
Chlamydia trachomatis (chlamydia)	
Neisseria gonorrhoeae (gonorrhea)	
Escherichia coli	

Referral

- Patients should be referred to urology or the ED depending on the severity of presentation and how well the patient responds treatment.

F. VARICOCELE

- A varicocele is an enlargement of the pampiniform venous plexus, the network of veins that drains the testicles.
- The pampiniform venous plexus is similar to the network of veins in the cardiovascular system as it has valves to prevent backflow.
- If one of the valves in the pampiniform venous plexus is defective, a varicocele occurs.
- Patients typically present without pain but may experience a dull ache or feeling of heaviness in the scrotum.
- Patients may describe a "bag-of-worms" sensation in the scrotum upon palpation.
- There is typically no trauma reported with this condition.

Diagnosis

- On physical exam, palpation will likely reveal a soft, boggy scrotum with a "bag-of-worms" feeling.

Treatment

- Treatment requires surgical correction.

Referral

- Patients must be referred to urology for surgical correction of the varicocele.

G. HYDROCELE

- A hydrocele is the collection of fluid around a testicle.
- There are four common causes of hydroceles (Table 13-4).

Treatment

- Treatment is via surgical repair.

Referral

- Patients should be referred to urology for surgical repair and management.

TABLE 13-4	The Four Common Causes of Hydroceles
Excessive production of fluid in the scrotum	
Altered fluid absorption	
Altered lymph drainage	
Hernia	

14

Obstetrics

Prenatal Care
   The Initial Prenatal Visit
   Medications and Substances to Avoid in Pregnancy
   Naegele's Rule
   Norms During Pregnancy
   Vaccines During Pregnancy
   Prenatal Appointments

Spontaneous Abortion

Ectopic Pregnancy

Third-Trimester Complications
   Placenta Previa
   Placental Abruption

Medical Conditions in Pregnancy
   Gestational Hypertension
   Gestational Diabetes

Postpartum Hemorrhage

Pre-eclampsia and Eclampsia

Gynecology

Routine Preventive Care

Menstruation Abnormalities
   Amenorrhea
   Dysmenorrhea
   Menorrhagia

Cervical Abnormalities

Breast Cancer

Breast Pain and Infection

Premenstrual Syndrome and Premenstrual Dysphoric Disorder
   Premenstrual Syndrome
   Premenstrual Dysphoric Disorder

The Menstrual Cycle

Contraception

Obstetrics

PRENATAL CARE

Case 1

A 25-year-old female pregnant for the first time (G1P0) presents to the office at 7 weeks' gestation. The patient has no relevant past medical history, no relevant past surgical history, and is taking no medications. She has intermittent nausea and vomiting, which resolve mostly on their own after eating.

Which of the following is included in the initial prenatal exam?

A. Maternal alpha-fetoprotein (MAFP) test

B. Oral glucose tolerance test

C. Pap smear

D. Chorionic villus sampling (CVS)

E. Group B *Streptococcus* testing

Discussion

The correct answer is C. You cannot do CVS or MAFP yet, because there is no routine indication for CVS in anyone and MAFP only has meaning once you are actually pregnant. The oral glucose tolerance test is not helpful because this test only becomes abnormal later in pregnancy when gestational diabetes is possible.

The Initial Prenatal Visit

The initial prenatal visit is very comprehensive and includes the following:

- Past medical history (PMH)
- Past surgical history (PSH)
- Assessment of allergies
- Assessment of medications
- Obstetric (OB) history (ie, how many previous pregnancies, abortions)
- Gynecological (GYN) history (including menstrual history)
- History of sexually transmitted diseases (STDs)
- Family history
- Social history

    Initial testing includes the following:

- Complete blood count (CBC)
- Complete metabolic profile (CMP)
- Thyroid profile
- Coombs testing
- Blood type
- Urinalysis (UA) and urine culture
- STD testing (chlamydia, gonorrhea, hepatitis, HIV, syphilis)
- Pap smear

    Testing that will be done at every visit includes the following:

- History
  - Contractions
  - Vaginal bleeding

TABLE 14-1	Fundal Height
NUMBER OF WEEKS OF GESTATION	**FUNDAL HEIGHT**
12	Symphysis pubis
16	Halfway between symphysis pubis and umbilicus
20	Level of umbilicus
24+	Number of weeks equals fundal height measured in centimeters

- Fluid leakage
- Fetal movements
■ Blood pressure (BP) monitoring
■ Weight monitoring
■ Fetal heart tones
■ Fundal height
  - Measures the uterus size.
  - Measurement is taken from the symphysis pubis to the top of the fundus (felt with hands).
  - Assesses fetal growth and development (ie, whether the fetus is too large or small for its gestational age).
  - Beginning in week 24, fundal height as measured in centimeters should be equal to gestational age (eg, for a gestational age of 25 weeks, the fundal height should be 25 cm) (Table 14-1).
■ Urine dipstick
  - Used to monitor for protein and glucose levels

Medications and Substances to Avoid During Pregnancy

The following medications and substances should be avoided during pregnancy:
■ Tamsulosin
■ Nonsteroidal anti-inflammatory drugs (NSAIDs), including acetylsalicylic acid (aspirin), ibuprofen, and naproxen (except in very specific circumstances)
■ Sulfa drugs
■ Lithium
■ Alcohol
■ Caffeine (Limit caffeine intake to less than 200 mg, or about 1 cup, per day)
■ Cigarettes

Naegele's Rule

■ Naegele's rule is used to estimate the date of delivery; however, it cannot be used for women with irregular menstrual cycles.
■ To use the rule, first subtract 3 months from the month of the mother's last menstrual period. Then add 7 days to the day of the mother's last menstrual period.

Norms During Pregnancy

■ Displacement of abdominal and chest organs upward and to the left to accommodate the growing fetus
■ Changes in thyroid function
■ Anemia and changes in plasma volume
■ Systolic murmur may develop as a result of increased blood volume
■ After 20 weeks' gestation, patients must be counseled to sleep on their side to avoid compression of the inferior vena cava
■ Decreased peristalsis causes constipation

- Relaxation of sphincters causes acid reflux
- Skin pigmentation changes as a result of hormonal changes

Vaccines During Pregnancy

Vaccines that should be administered during pregnancy include the following:

- Flu vaccine (during flu season)
- Tetanus, diphtheria, and pertussis (Tdap)
  - Tdap is administered during every pregnancy for acellular pertussis (whooping cough) protection and tetanus prevention.

Both vaccines may be administered postpartum but should be recommended during pregnancy.

Vaccines to be *avoided* during pregnancy include the following:

- Measles, mumps, and rubella (MMR)
- Rubella
- Varicella
- All live vaccines

Prenatal Appointments

Prenatal patients have appointments

- Every 4 weeks from the initial visit to 28 weeks
- Every 2 weeks from 28 weeks to 36 weeks
- Every week from 36 weeks to delivery

The 10-to-13-Week Visit

- The visit at 10-13 weeks is important in women who are considered to be of advanced maternal age, meaning over the age of 35.
- Women who are of advanced maternal age or who have an increased risk of passing on genetic diseases have the option to undergo CVS sampling.
  - CVS sampling is done to obtain a karyotype of the fetus in order to detect any chromosomal abnormalities.
  - CVS sampling is done by placing a long, thin needle through the abdomen into the placenta to obtain a sample of chorionic villi cells.
  - Complications of CVS sampling include fetal loss.
- Nuchal translucency (NT) is also done at 10-13 weeks (Figure 14-1).
  - NT involves an abdominal ultrasound, paying special attention to the neck.
  - If a nuchal translucency is present, there is an increased risk of Down syndrome.

CLINICAL TIP
The number of weeks of gestation determines the testing that should be done.

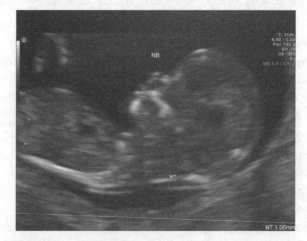

FIGURE 14-1 Nuchal translucency. Reproduced with permission from DeCherney AH, Nathan L, Laufer N: *Current Diagnosis & Treatment: Obstetrics & Gynecology*, 11th ed. New York, NY: McGraw-Hill; 2013.

Amniocentesis

- Amniocentesis is another test that can be performed to obtain the karyotype of the fetus.
- An amniocentesis is done between 15 and 20 weeks' gestation in women of advanced maternal age.
- An amniocentesis involves obtaining fluid from the amniotic sac.
- This is the recommended option for genetic screening as it has fewer associated fetal complications compared to chorionic villous sampling.

The 16-to-18-Week Visit

- The Maternal alpha-fetoprotein (MAFP) test is done at the visit at 16-18 weeks.
- The MAFP is part of either the triple screen (Table 14-2) or quad screen (Table 14-3).
- When MAFP results are abnormal—whether high or low—an ultrasound is required.
- The most common reason for an abnormal MAFP is an error in dating; the date of conception may be earlier or later than originally thought.
- A high MAFP level is common in twins, neural tube defects, abdominal wall defects, threatened abortion, or fetuses of more than 18 weeks' gestational age.
- A low MAFP level is common in Down syndrome and in fetuses of less than 16 weeks' gestational age.
- The ultrasound performed following abnormal MAFP results involves first visualizing the fetus. If the dating is correct and no structural abnormalities are seen, an amniocentesis should be recommended.

CLINICAL TIP
When MAFP results are abnormal, whether high or low, an ultrasound is required.

Visits Between 26 and 36 Weeks

- At one of the visits between 26 and 30 weeks, patients undergo the 1-hour oral glucose tolerance test (OGTT) to test for gestational diabetes (Table 14-4).
- The OGTT is done without fasting. The patient drinks a solution containing 50 g of glucose, and blood is drawn 1 hour later.
- If the patient's blood glucose level is more than 140 mg/dL, which suggests gestational diabetes, a 3-hour OGTT is performed to confirm gestational diabetes (Table 14-5).

TABLE 14-2	Triple Screen
Maternal alpha-fetoprotein (MAFP)	
Human chorionic gonadotropin (HCG)	
Estriol	

TABLE 14-3	Quad Screen
Maternal alpha-fetoprotein (MAFP)	
Human chorionic gonadotropin (HCG)	
Estriol	
Inhibin A	

TABLE 14-4	One-Hour Oral Glucose Tolerance Test
Performed nonfasting
Patient consumes 50 g of glucose
If blood glucose > 140 mg/dL, a 3-hour OGTT is performed.

TABLE 14-5	Three-Hour Oral Glucose Tolerance Test
Performed fasting
Fasting blood glucose level is measured
Patient consumes 100 g of glucose
Blood drawn at 1, 2, and 3 hours following glucose consumption
Blood glucose levels considered abnormally high: ■ Fasting: > 95 mg/dL ■ 1 hour: > 180 mg/dL ■ 2 hours: > 155 mg/dL ■ 3 hours: > 140 mg/dL
Two or more abnormally high levels confirm gestational diabetes.

CLINICAL TIP
- A 1-hour OGTT is used to screen for gestational diabetes.
- A 3-hour OGTT is used to confirm gestational diabetes.

- The 3-hour OGTT is done fasting.
- In the 3-hour OGTT, blood is drawn fasting (before the solution is consumed) and then 1, 2, and 3 hours following consumption of a solution containing 100 g of glucose. If at least 2 of the blood glucose levels drawn are abnormally high, the test is considered to be positive for gestational diabetes.

The 28-Week Visit

- The 28-week visit is important if the mother is Rh negative as this is the visit at which RhoGAM will be administered.
- When a woman is Rh negative and the infant's father is RH positive, there is a change that the infant will be Rh positive.
- RhoGAM is given to prevent any incompatibility of the Rh factor.
- Palpation of the gravid abdomen will also be done to determine if the baby is in breech presentation.

The 36-Week Visit

- The 36-week visit involves group B *Streptococcus* screening and obtaining vaginal and perirectal cultures to test for the presence of group A *Streptococcus*. This testing helps determine if the patient will need antibiotics during labor.
- Palpation and ultrasound will also be performed to determine whether the fetus is in breech presentation.

SPONTANEOUS ABORTION

Case 2

A 19-year-old female with an intrauterine pregnancy at 14 weeks presents to the emergency department (ED) for vaginal bleeding. The patient states that the bleeding started early that morning, that a moderate amount of blood has been lost, and that no clots have been seen. The patient states that there are no aggregating or alleviating factors.

TABLE 14-6	Types of Spontaneous Abortion	
TYPE OF SPONTANEOUS ABORTION	ULTRASOUND FINDINGS	TREATMENT
Complete abortion	Cervix is closed No products of conception are seen	No further treatment
Incomplete abortion	Some products of conception are seen in the uterus	D&C to cleanse the uterine lining
Threatened abortion	Normal pregnancy Closed cervical os	Close monitoring Bed rest
Inevitable abortion	Opened cervical os Signs of fetal distress: no movement, slow heart rate	Hospital admission OB/GYN consultation
Septic abortion	Retained products of conception Signs of bleeding and infection	Hospital admission Intravenous (IV) antibiotics Possible D&C

What is the next step in the management of this patient?

A. Continue to monitor for resolution

B. Beta-human chorionic gonadotropin (B-HCG) testing now and again in 48 hours

C. Ultrasound

D. Administer misoprostol

Discussion

The correct answer is C. The most common cause of vaginal bleeding in the first and second trimesters is spontaneous abortion. The type of spontaneous abortion can be determined only through ultrasound. Neither monitoring for resolution nor checking B-HCG will determine the type of abortion. Misoprostol induces abortion.

In addition to ultrasound, if the mother is Rh negative and the pregnancy is viable, RhoGAM should be administered. If ultrasound confirms spontaneous abortion, medical management may include the administration of misoprostol to aid in contractions to help remove the products of conception. Surgical intervention includes dilation and curettage (D&C).

The types of spontaneous abortion and their corresponding ultrasound findings and treatments are given in Table 14-6.

ECTOPIC PREGNANCY

Case 3

A 35-year-old female presents to the ED with significant right lower quadrant abdominal pain, which she describes as sharp, stabbing, and worsening. The pain is radiating to the patient's right shoulder. The patient describes her current menstruation as abnormal, with her last period having occurred 8 weeks ago. Her vitals are positive for elevated BP. Her physical exam is positive for right lower quadrant abdominal pain.

Which of the following is the next step in the management of this patient?

A. Abdominal ultrasound

B. Computerized tomography (CT) scan of abdomen and pelvis

C. Magnetic resonance imaging (MRI) of abdomen and pelvis

D. Urine B-HCG test

Discussion

The correct answer is D. An ectopic pregnancy is any pregnancy that occurs outside of the uterus. Ectopic pregnancies most commonly take place in the fallopian tubes. Once the fetus grows too large, it can cause a significant amount of pain and may rupture the tube if not caught early. Ectopic pregnancy most commonly presents with unilateral pelvic pain, which may radiate to the shoulders. The patient may or may not know she is pregnant; therefore, every woman of childbearing age who presents to the ED with unilateral pelvic pain should undergo a urine B-HCG test to determine which imaging test should be performed.

Ultrasound is the diagnostic test of choice if B-HCG is positive, as it is cheaper and more readily available than CT and also safe in pregnancy. A CT scan is performed for unilateral abdominal pain when B-HCG is negative to rule out appendicitis in right lower quadrant abdominal pain.

An MRI is not done as a screening test for ectopic pregnancy. A CBC will not determine the cause of unilateral abdominal pain but will indicate whether an infection is present.

CLINICAL TIP
Unilateral pelvic pain + positive B-HCG = ultrasound

THIRD-TRIMESTER COMPLICATIONS

Case 4

A 24-year-old female who is 34 weeks' pregnant presents with painless vaginal bleeding. BP is normal. There is no edema.

Which of the following is the most likely diagnosis?

A. Placenta previa

B. Placental abruption

C. Pre-eclampsia

D. Labor

Discussion

The correct answer is A. Placenta previa must always be ruled out in cases of painless vaginal bleeding in pregnancy after 20 weeks. Placental abruption is usually painful, as it involves the placenta being pulled away from the uterine wall. Labor would be associated with pain. Pre-eclampsia is associated with hypertension, edema and proteinuria.

Placenta Previa

- Placenta previa is the partial or full blockage of the cervical os by the placenta (Figure 14-2).
- In normal pregnancy, the placenta is implanted on the side wall of the uterine lining.
- There are several types of placenta previa:
  - Marginal: The placenta does not cover the internal cervical os but is very close to it.
  - Partial: The placenta partially covers the internal cervical os.
  - Complete: The placenta entirely covers the internal cervical os.
- In low-lying placenta, the placenta lies close to the internal cervical os but does not touch it.

Diagnosis

- Diagnosis is made via ultrasound to evaluate implantation site of the placenta.

Treatment

- Placenta previa patients are treated by obstetrician/gynecologists (OB/GYNs).
- Patients must be placed on immediate pelvic rest (nothing inserted into the vagina).

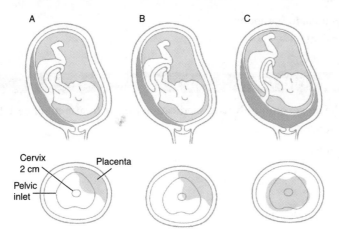

FIGURE 14-2 Types of Placental Disorders. Reproduced with permission from DeCherney AH, Nathan L, Laufer N: *Current Diagnosis & Treatment: Obstetrics & Gynecology*, 11th ed. New York, NY: McGraw-Hill; 2013.

Complications

- Placenta previa is a common cause of third-trimester vaginal bleeding.
- The vaginal bleeding typical of placenta previa is *painless*.
- If a pregnant patient presents with painless vaginal bleeding, an internal vaginal exam should *never* be done, as this can worsen bleeding if it is caused by placenta previa.

Placental Abruption

- Placental abruption occurs when the placenta pulls away from the uterine wall.
- Placental abruption usually occurs at 20 weeks' gestation or later.
- When the placenta pulls away from the uterine wall, *painful* vaginal bleeding occurs.
- Placental abruption is commonly caused by blunt trauma to the abdomen, such as in car accidents or falls.
- Patients typically present with a sudden onset of abdominal pain, painful vaginal bleeding, abdominal tenderness, syncope, decreased fetal movement, and fetal tachycardia.
- This condition has several maternal and fetal implications (Table 14-7).

Diagnosis

- Diagnosis is made via ultrasound, which will demonstrate the placenta pulling away from the uterine wall.

Risk Factors

- Maternal hypertension
- Maternal cocaine use

CLINICAL TIP

Women with placenta previa typically deliver by Caesarean section (C-section) unless the placenta is positioned at least 2 cm away from the internal cervical os.

CLINICAL TIP

Never do an internal exam in a patient with *painless* vaginal bleeding in third trimester.

CLINICAL TIP

In placenta previa, patients must be advised that *nothing* is to be inserted into the vagina.

TABLE 14-7	Maternal and Fetal Implications of Placental Abruption	
MATERNAL IMPLICATIONS	FETAL IMPLICATIONS
Tachycardia	Loss of blood supply
Volume loss	Loss of nutrients
Syncope	
Severe anemia	

- Blunt trauma to the abdomen
- Car accident

MEDICAL CONDITIONS IN PREGNANCY

What is the most commonly used medication for the treatment of gestational hypertension?

A. Metoprolol

B. Labetalol

C. Losartan

D. Hydrochlorothiazide

Discussion

The correct answer is B. Labetalol is the most commonly used medication used for gestational hypertension. Metoprolol, losartan, and hydrochlorothiazide are not used in the management of gestational hypertension ACE inhibitors and angiotensin receptor blockers like losartan are contraindicated. Although metoprolol, like all beta blockers, is safe to use in pregnancy. It is just not as effective. Diuretics may be associated with decreased fetal size by pulling perfusion away from the fetus.

Gestational Hypertension

- Gestational hypertension is hypertension that occurs in pregnant women after 20 weeks of gestation.
- If hypertension is diagnosed prior to 20 weeks' gestation, it is considered overt hypertension.

Risk Factors

- Obesity
- Advanced maternal age (over 35)
- Previous diagnosis of hypertension
- Previous diagnosis of diabetes
- Multiple gestation (eg, twins)

Diagnosis

- Gestational hypertension is diagnosed based on blood pressure readings of above 140/90 mm Hg on 2 separate occasions 2 or more weeks apart.

Treatment

- Lifestyle modifications are first line treatment: decrease salt intake and engage in low-impact cardiovascular exercises.
- Medications for hypertension in pregnancy include labetalol (most commonly used),calcium channel blockers, methyldopa, or hydralazine.

Referral

- The OB/GYN should be involved in all aspects of patient care.
- Patients may be referred back to the primary care nurse practitioner for medication management.

Gestational Diabetes

- Gestational diabetes is a condition in which women who have not previously been diagnosed with diabetes exhibit elevated blood glucose levels during pregnancy.

Diagnosis

- Diagnosis of gestational diabetes is based on a hemoglobin A1c (HbA1c) level greater than 6.5%.
- The 3-hour OGTT is also used to diagnose gestational diabetes (see Table 14-5).

CLINICAL TIP

Hypertension is diagnosed when blood pressure is higher than 140/90 mm Hg.

CLINICAL TIP

If protein or edema is present, a diagnosis of pre-eclampsia is considered.

Risk Factors

- Polycystic ovary syndrome (PCOS)
- History of prediabetes
- Family history of diabetes
- Maternal age (35+)
- African American ethnicity
- Obesity

Treatment

- Treatment is similar to that for type 2 diabetes mellitus.
- Lifestyle modifications comprise first-line treatment: gentle, low-impact cardiovascular exercise (taking precautions to protect the fetus) and a low-carbohydrate diet.
- Metformin is the primary oral therapy.
- Insulin is used if lifestyle modifications and oral therapy fail.

Complications

- Large baby
- Delivery complications, such as shoulder dystocia, due to baby's size
- Complications for baby following delivery (eg, hypoglycemia)

Referral

- Patients should be closely monitored by an OB/GYN.
- An endocrinology consultation may be considered if there is difficulty with glucose control.

CLINICAL AND EXAM TIP
Gestational diabetes is associated with the development of type 2 diabetes later in life.

POSTPARTUM HEMORRHAGE

- Postpartum hemorrhage is defined as losing more than 1 L (1000 mL) of blood during or up to 1 day after delivery.

Risk Factors

- History of coagulopathy
- Poor uterine contraction
- Retained placenta
- Presence of anemic pre-delivery
- C-section delivery

Diagnosis

- Diagnosis is based on the large amount of vaginal bleeding.
- Patients may also experience tachycardia, dizziness, and fatigue.

Treatment

- Treatment is typically addressed in the in-patient setting.
- If the patient has already returned home, immediate transportation back to hospital is required for appropriate in-patient treatment.
- Treatment consists of IV fluids and medications such as oxytocin to induce uterine contraction.

PRE-ECLAMPSIA AND ECLAMPSIA

- Pre-eclampsia is a condition characterized by hypertension, proteinuria (a large amount of protein in the urine), and edema. Pre-eclampsia usually occurs in the third trimester of pregnancy.
- Eclampsia is the onset of seizures in a woman with pre-eclampsia.

CLINICAL TIP
Pre-eclampsia + seizures = eclampsia

Complications

- Fetal and maternal oxygen deprivation
- Aspiration
- Cerebral damage
- Hemorrhage

Diagnosis

A diagnosis of pre-eclampsia is based on the following:

- Blood pressure > 140/90 mm Hg
- Urine protein reading of 3+
- Presence of edema

A diagnosis of eclampsia is made when a patient with pre-eclampsia suffers a seizure.

Risk Factors

- Pre-existing hypertension
- Pre-existing diabetes
- Large placenta
- History of coagulopathy

Treatment of Pre-eclampsia

- Patients with pre-eclampsia are treated by an OB/GYN.
- Labetalol is commonly used to treat hypertension and control blood pressure in pre-eclampsia.
- Magnesium sulfate is given to prevent seizures.
- Pre-eclampsia patients are often placed on bed rest.

Referral

- Patients must be promptly referred to an OB/GYN.

CLINICAL AND EXAM TIP
In pregnant patients with edema, always check for elevated blood pressure and proteinuria.

Gynecology

ROUTINE PREVENTIVE CARE

- Pap smears begin at age 21 regardless of sexual activity.
  - Pap smears stop at age 65.
- Breast screening begins at age 50.
  - In cases of a first-degree relative with breast cancer, screening begins 10 years before the age of the youngest relative at diagnosis.
  - Routine breast screening stops at age 70.

MENSTRUATION ABNORMALITIES

A. Amenorrhea

- Amenorrhea is the absence of menstruation.
- Amenorrhea can be primary or secondary.
- The most common cause of primary amenorrhea is pregnancy.
- The most common cause of secondary amenorrhea is hormonal abnormalities.
- A decrease in body fat, as often occurs in athletes, and anorexia can cause secondary amenorrhea.
- In cases of amenorrhea, ensure no chronic condition, such as Turner syndrome, or other endocrine abnormalities are present (eg, hirsutism, acne, male pattern balding, obesity, lack of secondary sexual characteristics).

Diagnostic Tests

- Pregnancy testing to rule out pregnancy
- Hormonal testing to rule out hormone-secreting tumors (pituitary or adrenal tumors)
  - Thyroid-stimulating hormone (TSH)
  - Follicle-stimulating hormone (FSH)
  - Luteinizing hormone (LH)

Referral

- In cases of secondary amenorrhea, patients should be referred to endocrinology.

B. Dysmenorrhea

- Dysmenorrhea is painful menstruation.
- Dysmenorrhea can be primary or secondary.
- Primary dysmenorrhea begins shortly after menarche.
- Secondary dysmenorrhea begins later in life.
- Pain may occur in the lower abdomen, low back, or flanks.
- Other symptoms include nausea, vomiting, fatigue, gastrointestinal discomfort, headache, and dizziness.

Diagnosis

- A clinical diagnosis is based on the presence of symptoms during menstruation.

Treatment

- The primary treatment of dysmenorrhea is an NSAID (eg, naproxen, ibuprofen).
- If persistent, oral hormonal birth control medications may be used to control menstruation.

CLINICAL TIP

For younger females, mammograms may not always produce the best images because of the density of the breast tissue. However, you will never be faulted, in real life or on the exam, for ordering mammography for a breast complaint.

CLINICAL TIP

Undiagnosed breast cancer is the most frequent reason for medical litigation.

CLINICAL TIP

In dysmenorrhea, an infectious origin (eg, pelvic inflammatory disease [PID], urinary tract infection [UTI]) and ectopic pregnancy must be ruled out.

Referral

- An OB/GYN referral can be made if the condition persists.
- OB/GYN consultations should also be considered for routine evaluation and if any concerning features present during physical evaluation.

C. Menorrhagia

- Menorrhagia is exceptionally heavy and prolonged bleeding during menstruation.
- Clotting may be present.
- Menorrhagia is usually without cause but can be secondary to miscarriage, endometriosis, uterine fibroids, or coagulopathy.

CLINICAL TIP
Menorrhagia can be associated with dysmenorrhea.

Diagnosis

- Diagnosis is based on the presence of menstrual bleeding that is heavier and of longer duration than usual.

Treatment

- The treatment of menorrhagia is similar to that for dysmenorrhea.
- The primary treatment of dysmenorrhea is an NSAID (eg, naproxen, ibuprofen).
- If persistent, oral hormonal birth control medications may be used to control menstruation.

CLINICAL AND EXAM TIP
Ensure patients with menorrhagia do not become anemic.

Referral

- An OB/GYN referral can be made if the condition persists.
- An OB/GYN consultation should also be considered for routine evaluation and if any concerning features present during physical evaluation.

CERVICAL ABNORMALITIES

- Cervical abnormalities range from benign to infectious to malignant (cancerous).
- The primary care nurse practitioner must perform routine Pap smears and gynecological evaluations on their female patients or ensure they are being completed by another healthcare professional.
- Cervical infections may present as UTIs with dysuria, urinary frequency, or urgency.
- Vaginal discharge may be present.

Diagnosis

- Pap smear
- Swab for culture and sensitivity
- Swab for herpes and human papillomavirus (HPV)

Treatment

- Treatment depends on the cause of the cervical abnormality.
- The antibiotics most commonly given include the following:
  - Ceftriaxone (if gonorrhea is suspected)
  - Azithromycin (if chlamydia is suspected)
  - Cephalexin and ciprofloxacin (commonly given for bacterial infections of the lower urinary tract)
  - Nitrofurantoin (commonly used in pregnant women)

CLINICAL TIP
Cases of lower urinary tract and genital infection in pregnancy should be referred to an OB/GYN.

Referral

- Primary care nurse practitioners typically refer patients to a women's health nurse practitioner or OB/GYN provider even though they are often the ones who perform the initial Pap smear and culture.

BREAST CANCER

Breast cancer is discussed in greater depth in Chapter 9.

- There are various presentations of breast cancer, ranging from the subtle (eg, mild change in shape or rash) to the obvious (eg, breast mass, nipple discharge).
- There are often genetic components to breast cancer, as with other cancers.
- It is imperative to evaluate *all* breast complaints for breast cancer.

BREAST PAIN AND INFECTION

- Breast pain and infections are very common presentations to primary care.
- Pain can be closely linked with menstruation.
- Common skin infections include erythema, which presents like cellulitis (see Chapter 15).
- Treatment for skin infection is the same as for cellulitis of any other body site, unless infection is thought to extend to deeper tissues.
- If nipple discharge is present, culture and sensitivity should be obtained to detect the presence of infection.
- In cases of breast pain, patients typically present with unilateral breast pain.

Diagnosis

- A physical exam is performed, checking for nipple inversion, discharge, the presence of a mass, or textured skin ("peau d'orange").

Treatment

- Breast pain is often treated with an NSAID (eg, naproxen, ibuprofen).
- Cellulitis of the breast tissue is treated with common oral antibiotics (eg, cephalexin, doxycycline).

Tests

- If clinically indicated, a culture and sensitivity of tissue and/or discharge may be evaluated.
- Breast mammography or ultrasonography may be performed.
- Core biopsy is also useful.

Referral

- Referral to OB/GYN or breast surgery is very useful if there is any cause for concern; for example, nonhealing wounds, continued pain, lymph nodes present, or any clinical features that indicate deeper infection.

CLINICAL TIP
Don't forget a chaperone who is a third party present during a breast or pelvic exam.

PREMENSTRUAL SYNDROME AND PREMENSTRUAL DYSPHORIC DISORDER

Case 5

A 22-year-old female with a history of premenstrual syndrome (PMS) presents, stating that she has started to experience worsening anxiety and depression just before her menstrual cycle begins. She reports having felt suicidal last month but that those thoughts resolved when menses stopped.

What is the best course of action?

A. Reassure the patient

B. Psychiatry referral

C. Start treatment with a selective serotonin reuptake inhibitor (SSRI)

D. OB/GYN referral

TABLE 14-8	Signs and Symptoms of Premenstrual Syndrome
Acne	
Breast tenderness	
Bloating	
Fatigue	
Irritability	
Mood changes	
Abdominal discomfort	

Discussion

The correct answer is B. While all options are logical choices, referring the patient to a psychiatrist to evaluate whether there are any nonorganic concerns and to monitor for further suicidal behaviors is paramount. If the patient is deemed to be actively suicidal, an ED referral should be completed—this is not an option here. Reassurance should be given, but that is not enough in cases of suicidal ideation. No medications should be prescribed until a full evaluation is completed.

Premenstrual Syndrome

- Premenstrual syndrome (PMS) is a complex combination of emotional and physical complaints that occur just prior to menstruation (Table 14-8).
- Symptoms usually resolve when menstruation completes.

Premenstrual Dysphoric Disorder

- Premenstrual dysphoric disorder (PMDD) is a severe form of PMS that affects less than 10% of the population (Table 14-9).
- PMDD occurs during the luteal phase of the menstrual cycle (see "The Menstrual Cycle").
- PMDD interferes with activities of daily living.

Diagnosis

- Diagnosis can be made via careful history by the primary care nurse practitioner when symptoms occur just prior to menstruation.

Treatment

- Lifestyle modifications can help relieve minor signs and symptoms of PMS and PMDD (eg, reduce salt and caffeine intake and increase exercise).

TABLE 14-9	Signs and Symptoms of Premenstrual Dysphoric Disorder
All signs and symptoms of PMDD	
Anxiety	
Depression	
Panic attacks	
Mood swings	
Fatigue	
Insomnia	
Suicidal thoughts	

- Stress reduction techniques, such as deep breathing exercises and yoga, may also help.
- SSRIs, such as fluoxetine or sertraline, may be used for severe PMS or PMDD.
- Oral hormonal contraceptives may be used to help modulate and regulate menstruation to reduce symptom severity.

Referral

- An OB/GYN referral should be made to rule out underlying causes and to ensure all relevant testing is performed (eg, Pap smear is up to date, a hormone evaluation is completed).
- In cases of PMDD, a psychiatry evaluation can be completed, especially if the patient is experiencing severe depression or anxiety.

CLINICAL TIP

If suicidal ideation is present, special precautions *must* be put into place: ED evaluation or other precautions to ensure the patient does not harm herself.

THE MENSTRUAL CYCLE

- The menstrual cycle is the hormonal exchange through which an ovum (egg) passes from the ovary down the fallopian tube to the uterus (Figure 14-3). If the egg becomes fertilized by a sperm, the woman becomes pregnant.
- The menstrual cycle is a complex process that usually begins around age 12. If it has yet to start by age 16, hormonal studies are conducted to rule out hormonal imbalances or other disease processes.
- The ovarian cycle consists of the follicular phase, ovulation, and the luteal phase (Table 14-10).

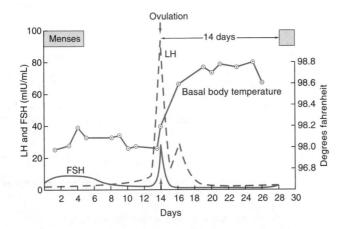

FIGURE 14-3 Hormone And Temperature Levels During A Normal Menstrual Cycle. Reproduced with permission from DeCherney AH, Nathan L, Laufer N: *Current Diagnosis & Treatment: Obstetrics & Gynecology*, 11th ed. New York, NY: McGraw-Hill; 2013.

TABLE 14-10	The Ovarian Cycle	
FOLLICULAR PHASE	**OVULATION**	**LUTEAL PHASE**
First stage of the menstrual cycle	Mature ovum is secreted	Final phase of the ovarian cycle
Follicle matures and releases an ovum	Estradiol increases level of luteinizing hormone (LH)	FSH and LH remain
Increase in follicle-stimulating hormone (FSH) level	Left and right ovaries take turns month to month	Hormones are required to maintain the ovum
Only one follicle per month becomes mature (and contains the ovum)		If the ovum is fertilized, human chorionic gonadotropic (hCG) is produced to protect the ovum

TABLE 14-11	The Uterine Cycle	
MENSTRUATION	PROLIFERATION	SECRETORY PHASE
First phase of uterine cycle	Corresponds with the luteal phase	Final phase of the uterine cycle
Sign that a woman is not pregnant	Progesterone increases	Allows the inner lining of the uterus to be renewed in preparation for the next month's cycle
Usually lasts 3-5 days	Implantation occurs if ovum is fertilized	
Abdominal or back cramping is common, as well as vaginal bleeding		

CLINICAL TIP

Menarche is the initial menstrual cycle. Menopause is the termination of the menstrual cycle.

CLINICAL TIP

Fertility occurs around day 14 of the menstrual cycle, during the luteal phase. Hormonal birth control (whether oral, topical, intravaginal, or injectable) works by interfering with this process.

- The uterine cycle consists of menstruation, proliferation, and the secretory phase (Table 14-11).

Contraception

- Methods of contraception are presented in Table 14-12.
- The choice of birth control method is a highly individual decision, based on the patient's personal preference and lifestyle needs.

TABLE 14-12	Methods of Contraception	
TYPE OF PROTECTION	COMMON BRAND NAMES	RISK FACTORS
Condom (male and female)	Durex, Lifestyles, Trojan	Allergic reaction Can break Ineffective if not properly applied
Oral hormonal agent (all involve either estrogen or progesterone or some combination thereof)	Gildess, Ortho Tri-Cyclen, TriNessa, Yaz	Blood clots (deep vein thrombosis [DVT] or pulmonary embolism [PE]); risk increased in smokers Ineffective if not taken regularly
Topical hormonal agent	Ortho Evra, Xulane	Skin irritation Patches have a higher concentration of estrogen than oral hormonal agents
Injectable hormonal agent	Depo-Provera	Weight gain Difficulty conceiving after discontinuation of therapy Injection site pain Allergic reaction
Intravaginal hormonal agent	NuvaRing	Allergic reaction Loss of ring
Intrauterine device (IUD)	Liletta, Mirena, ParaGard (copper based), Skyla	Can puncture uterine wall String can become lost Scarring of uterine wall

15
Dermatology

A. RASHES

AA. Pityriasis Rosea

- Pityriasis rosea is a viral rash characterized by a single erythematous lesion, referred to as a "herald patch," followed a diffuse body rash of small erythematous lesions lasting 6-12 weeks (Figure 15-1).
- Patients may present with upper respiratory infection–like signs and symptoms preceding the rash.

Diagnosis

- It is important to rule out other conditions such as fungal infections, Lyme disease, and other infections.

Treatment

- There is no specific therapy since the condition is usually self-limited.
- Treatment is for symptom management; antipruritics are often used, and topical steroids may be used if there is a lot of itching.
- UV light may help resolve the lesions.

CLINICAL TIP
Pityriasis rosea is also known as a "Christmas tree" rash.

CLINIC AND EXAM TIP
When you think about pityriasis rosea, think "herald rash" and "Christmas tree rash."

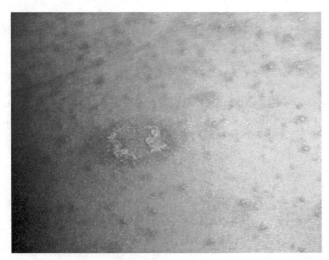

FIGURE 15-1 Pityriasis Rosea. Used with permission from Berger TG, Dept. Dermatology, UCSF.

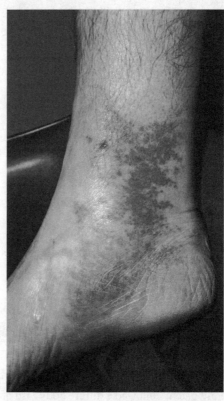

FIGURE 15-2　Dermatologic Disorders. Used with permission from Berger TG, Dept. Dermatology, UCSF.

AB. Cellulitis

- Cellulitis is a bacterial skin infection involving the top three layers of skin: the epidermis, dermis, and subcutaneous fat (Figure 15-2).
- Cellulitis is defined as an area of erythema that increases in size over a period of days.
- Erysipelas is a skin infection that affects only the epidermis and dermis layers, which are more superficial than the subcutaneous tissues.

Diagnosis

- A diagnosis of cellulitis is made clinically, based on how the condition looks; there is no specific imaging test to diagnose cellulitis.
- The affected area can be any size or shape anywhere on the body.
- Cellulitis will appear red and will feel warm and tender to palpation.
- A specific organism is rarely diagnosed, as there is no easy way to obtain a specific organism from the skin. Because of this, treatment is empirical, based on the organisms found most commonly in the past.

Treatment

Minor Cellulitis

- Oral cephalexin or dicloxacillin
- Oral therapy for methicillin-resistant *Staphylococcus aureus* (MRSA):
  - Sulfamethoxazole/trimethoprim
  - Clindamycin
  - Doxycycline
  - Linezolid

CLINICAL TIP

Cellulitis-causing bacteria often enter the skin through pimples, scratches, and other breaks in the skin.

CLINICAL TIP

Common bacterial causes of cellulitis infection are *Streptococcus pyogenes* and *Staphylococcus aureus*.

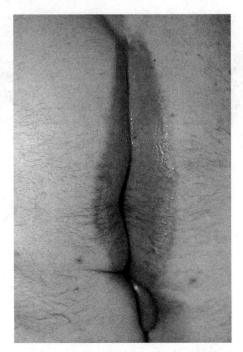

FIGURE 15-3 Intertrigo. Reproduced with permission from Wolff K, Johnson R, Saavedra AP: *Fitzpatrick's Color Atlas and Synopsis of Clinical Dermatology*, 7th ed. New York, NY: McGraw-Hill; 2013.

Severe Cellulitis

Severe cellulitis requires intravenous (IV) therapy:

- Cefazolin
- Vancomycin
- Ceftaroline (the only cephalosporin that covers MRSA)

AC. Intertrigo

- Intertrigo is an inflammatory rash of skin folds that is of bacterial, viral, or fungal origin (Figure 15-3).

Diagnosis

- Diagnosis is based on the clinical impression and the location of the rash.
- It is important to determine the underlying cause of the rash, as this will guide treatment.

Treatment

- Barrier creams are used to prevent inflammation and infection spread.
- The underlying cause of the infection must be treated.

AD. Vitiligo

- Vitiligo is a chronic skin condition characterized by changes in pigment (as a result of nonfunctional pigment cells or pigment cell death) (Figure 15-4).

Diagnosis

- Vitiligo is easily assessed as the patient will have patches of unpigmented skin.
- This change in skin pigmentation is the only diagnostic test for vitiligo.

Treatment

- There is no treatment for vitiligo.
- Cosmetics and depigmentation of the remaining pigmented skin may be used to help the patient feel more comfortable.

CLINICAL AND EXAM TIP
- Cellulitis can occur on any area of the body.
- The affected area will be red, warm, and painful to palpation.
- Use caution to ensure the infection does not appear to be spreading.
- Cellulitis around the eye is a *medical emergency*.

CLINICAL TIP
Common intertrigo sites include abdominal folds, the area under the breasts, inguinal areas, the buttocks, and behind the ears.

CLINICAL TIP
- There is a higher risk of intertrigo among individuals who have undergone amputation, those with diabetes, those who use diapers, and those on bed rest.
- Appearance is based on the causative factor: bacterial infections will look like cellulitis, and fungal infections will appear erythematous and scaly.

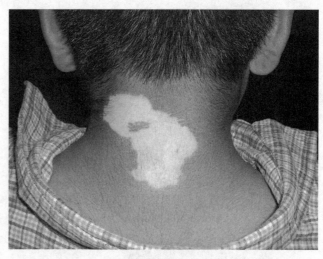

FIGURE 15-4 Vitiligo. Reproduced with permission from Richard P. Usatine, MD and Usatine RP, Smith MA, Chumley HS, et al: *The Color Atlas of Family Medicine*, 2nd ed. New York, NY: McGraw-Hill; 2013.

AE. Impetigo

- Impetigo is a contagious skin infection seen commonly in preschool-aged children (Figure 15-5).
- Contact sports increase risk of this condition.
- Bullous impetigo is characterized by fluid-filled blisters surrounded by erythema; when the blisters break, yellow scabs result.
- Impetigo can lead to post-*Streptococcal* glomerulonephritis.
- Impetigo does not cause rheumatic fever.

Diagnosis

- Diagnosis is made based on the presence of honey-colored scabs around erythematous lesions.

Treatments

- Treatment consists of oral antibiotics such as cephalexin, erythromycin, and sulfamethoxazole/trimethoprim.
- Topical antibiotics, such as bacitracin, retapamulin, or mupirocin, may also be used.

CLINICAL TIP
Honey-colored crusting is the hallmark of impetigo.

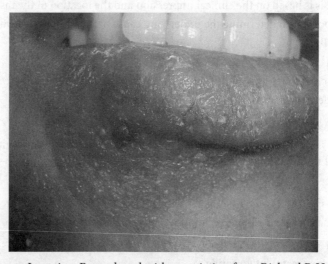

FIGURE 15-5 Impetigo. Reproduced with permission from Richard P. Usatine, MD and Usatine RP, Smith MA, Chumley HS, et al: *The Color Atlas of Family Medicine*, 2nd ed. New York, NY: McGraw-Hill; 2013.

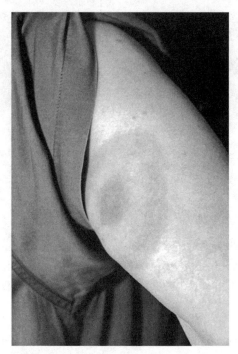

FIGURE 15-6 Lyme Disease. Used with permission from James Gathany, Public Health Image Library, CDC.

AF. Lyme Disease

- Lyme disease is a bacterial infection caused by *Borrelia* bacteria (Figure 15-6).
- Lyme disease is spread by infected ticks of the *Ixodes* genus.
- There is no such entity as chronic Lyme disease.

Signs and Symptoms

- The signs and symptoms of Lyme disease are presented in Table 15-1.

Diagnosis

- Patients must be carefully evaluated for signs of erythema migrans (the "bulls-eye" rash).
- Patients in later stages presenting with joint pain, neurological involvement, or cardiac involvement need laboratory testing.
- Lyme disease is confirmed with an enzyme-linked immunosorbent assay (ELISA), western blot test, or polymerase chain reaction (PCR) test.

Treatment

- Antibiotics, such as doxycycline, amoxicillin, or cefuroxime, are first-line therapy for involvement of the skin, joints, or facial palsy.
- Doxycycline is not used in patients under 8 years of age.

CLINICAL AND EXAM TIP
Erythema migrans, a spreading of erythema, is a key characteristic of early-stage Lyme disease; it is often referred to as the "bull's eye" rash.

TABLE 15-1	Signs and Symptoms of Lyme Disease	
EARLY INFECTION	**DISSEMINATED INFECTION**	**LATE STAGES OF INFECTION**
Erythema migrans (the "bull's eye" rash): erythematous, circular rash with central clearing Flu-like symptoms: weakness, malaise, headache, fever	Muscle tone changes Neurologic signs such as facial palsy	Joint pain (most common long-term complication) Atrioventricular (AV) block (most common form of cardiac involvement)

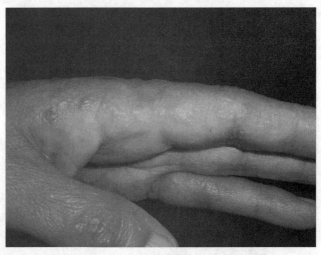

FIGURE 15-7 Eczema. Reproduced with permission from Richard P. Usatine, MD and Usatine RP, Smith MA, Chumley HS, et al: *The Color Atlas of Family Medicine*, 2nd ed. New York, NY: McGraw-Hill; 2013.

- Cefuroxime or amoxicillin can be used in children for Lyme disease that involves the skin, joints, or facial palsy.
- Ceftriaxone is used for nervous system Lyme disease (Lyme disease affecting the central nervous system [CNS]) and Lyme carditis (Lyme disease affecting the heart).

Referral

- An infectious disease consultation should be considered for this condition.

AG. Eczema

- Eczema (atopic dermatitis) is an inflammatory condition of the skin that is characterized by erythema, pruritis, and crusty patches (Figure 15-7).
- "Eczema" and "atopic dermatitis" are synonymous.

Signs and Symptoms

- Erythematous, swollen skin
- Pruritis
- Dry skin with flaking or crusting
- More severe: cracking, oozing, and bleeding skin

Diagnosis

- Diagnosis is based on a physical exam revealing the skin symptoms described above; this is the only method of diagnosing eczema.

Treatment

- Hygiene, moisturizing agents, antihistamines, and topical steroids are common in the treatment of eczema.
- The antihistamines used include loratadine, fexofenadine, and cetirizine.
- In severe cases, phototherapy or topical immunosuppressants may be indicated.
- The topical immunosuppressants used include tacrolimus, sirolimus, andcyclosporine, all of which inhibit T-cell function.

Referral

- Referral to dermatology is indicated if the eczema is severe, refractory, or diffuse.

AH. Psoriasis

- Psoriasis is a chronic inflammatory skin condition (Figure 15-8).
- Psoriasis is characterized by erythematous scaly areas called plaques.
- Pruritis is commonly present.

CLINICAL TIP
Food allergies or intolerances and drug allergies can produce eczema-like symptoms.

CLINICAL TIP
Eczema is more common in younger people and can be outgrown.

CLINICAL TIP
Extensor surfaces are commonly affected in psoriasis: the scalp, palms of hands, soles of feet, elbows, and knees.

CLINICAL TIP
Psoriasis is thought to be immune mediated.

CLINICAL TIP
Psoriasis can cause arthritis.

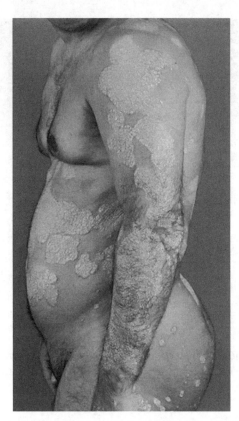

FIGURE 15-8 Psoriasis. Reproduced with permission from Wolff K, Johnson R, Suurmond, R: *Fitzpatrick's Color Atlas & Synopsis of Clinical Dermatology*, 5th ed. New York, NY: McGraw-Hill; 2005.

Diagnosis

- In most cases, skin appearance alone is sufficient to establish a diagnosis.

Treatment

- Topical steroids are first-line therapy.
- Topical salicylic acid may also used to decrease skin inflammation.
- Chronic steroids use can cause skin atrophy.
- Vitamin A and D derivatives help ease patients off steroids.
- When the disease is too widespread to cover with topical steroids or immunosuppressants, ultraviolet light is used.
- Those not controlled with ultraviolet light are treated with tumor necrosis factor (TNF) inhibitors such as adalimumab, etanercept, or infliximab.
- In severe cases, systemic oral medications, such as methotrexate are used to suppress the immune system. Since methotrexate causes liver and lung fibrosis, this is always the last choice for treatment when other therapies fail.

Referral

- A referral to dermatology may be indicated for refractory or resistant psoriasis.

AI. Seborrheic Dermatitis

- Seborrheic dermatitis is a chronic mild inflammation of the skin (Figure 15-9).
- Seborrheic dermatitis is a hypersensitivity reaction of the skin to fungus in the skin.
- Because of the hypersensitivity reaction and fungal involvement, both antifungal medications and steroids are effective in treatment.

CLINICAL AND EXAM TIP
Be aware that psoriasis can become systemic and affect more than the skin.

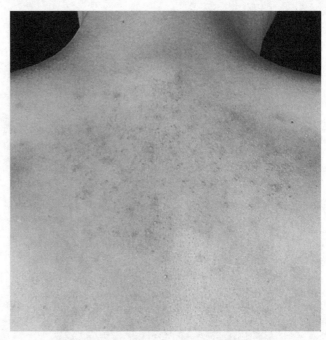

FIGURE 15-9 Acne. Reproduced with permission from Goldsmith LA, Katz S, Gilchrest B: *Fitzpatrick's Dermatology in General Medicine*, 8th ed. New York, NY: McGraw-Hill; 2012.

- In the infant population, the condition is also known as cradle cap.
- In the pediatric population, there is an oily, yellow crust around the scalp.
- Seborrheic dermatitis affects areas of the skin that have a high concentration of sebaceous glands such as the scalp, face, and torso.
- Hair loss from the affected areas may also occur.

Diagnosis

- The diagnosis of seborrheic dermatitis includes the presentation of skin areas that are scaly, flaky, itchy, and erythematous.

Treatment

- Topical steroids are used to reduce inflammation.
- If a fungal origin is suspected, topical antifungals, such as nystatin, clotrimazole, or ketoconazole, are used.
- Terbinafine is also used as a topical agent.
- If pruritis is present, antipruritics, such as antihistamines, may be given orally or topically.

AJ. Acne

- Acne is a chronic skin condition characterized by greasy skin, black heads, white heads, and, in severe cases, nodules and scars from these lesions (Figure 15-10).
- The sebaceous glands appear to be overactive in this condition.
- Sex hormones have a role in this process.
- Acne is more prevalent in the teenage years when sex hormones appear.
- The sebaceous glands have testosterone receptors and that is why there is more acne at the time of puberty.

Diagnosis

- The diagnosis of acne is based on the presentation of greasy skin, comedones, papules, pustules, and/or nodules along the face, chest, back, and/or neck.

CLINICAL TIP

Hygiene habits do not have an influence on acne.

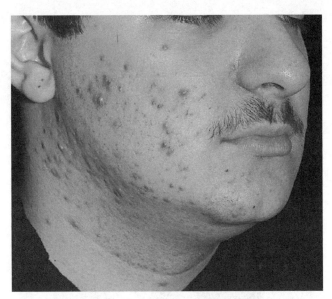

FIGURE 15-10 Comedones of acne. Reproduced with permission from Wolff K, Johnson R, Saavedra AP. eds. *Fitzpatrick's Color Atlas and Synopsis of Clinical Dermatology*, 7th ed. New York, NY: McGraw-Hill; 2013.

Treatment

- First-line therapy consists of topical treatments such as the following:
  - Benzoyl peroxide
  - Topical antibiotics (eg, erythromycin, clindamycin)
  - Topical salicylic acid if benzoyl peroxide and topical antibiotics are ineffective
  - Topical vitamin A (eg, retinoids)
- If topical therapy is ineffective, oral antibiotics, such as doxycycline or minocycline, are used.
- Spironolactone is effective in women to treat hirsutism associated with acne.
- For refractive acne and for nodular acne, isotretinoin may be given.
  - Isotretinoin is a category X medication: not for use in pregnancy.
  - For isotretinoin to be initiated, patients must agree to use two forms of birth control methods (eg, abstinence; oral, intramuscular, or intravaginal hormonal therapy; barrier methods such as male or female condoms).

Referral

- Initial acne treatments may be initiated by the primary care nurse practitioner.
- If initial treatments fail to be effective, a dermatology referral may be given.

B. SKIN CANCER

BA. Basal Cell Carcinoma

- Basal cell carcinoma is a common cancer.
- This cancer rarely spreads to other areas and rarely causes death.
- Caucasians are the most common group of people to be affected by basal cell carcinoma.
- Basal cell carcinoma presents as a pearly, shiny skin nodule or red area that has thickened (Figure 15-11).

Diagnosis

- Diagnosis is confirmed by biopsy.

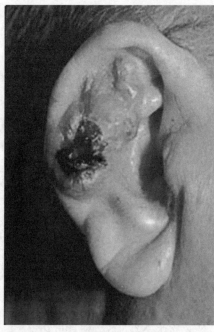

FIGURE 15-11 Basal cell cancer needs biopsy and removal. Reproduced with permission from Bondi EE, Jegasothy BV, Lazarus GS: *Dermatology Diagnosis and Therapy*, 1st ed. Norwalk, CT: Appleton & Lange; 1991.

Treatment

- Treatment involves surgical removal of the lesion, either through tradition surgical techniques or cryosurgery.
- Topical chemotherapeutic agents, such as 5-fluorouracil, may be used.
- Radiation therapy may also be used.

Referral

- If basal cell carcinoma is suspected, the patient should be referred to dermatology.

BB. Squamous Cell Carcinoma

- Squamous cell carcinoma is characterized by a multiplication of epithelial cells.
- Squamous cell carcinoma commonly appears among individuals in their 50s.
- Squamous cell carcinoma results from exposure to direct sunlight without protection.
- Squamous cell carcinoma presents as an ulcer or reddened area on the affected area of skin (Figure 15-12).
- An area of ulceration is commonly the presenting skin area.
- An ulceration that bleeds and fails to heal is a common skin complaint.

Diagnosis

- Skin biopsy is the definitive diagnostic tool.

Treatment

- Treatment consists of surgical removal of the lesion.
- Radiotherapy may be used.
- There is very little effective chemotherapy for either squamous cell carcinoma or basal cell carcinoma. Only for melanoma is chemotherapy meaningfully effective. Treatment for most skin cancers comes down to two words: biopsy and remove.

CLINICAL TIP
Patients with fair skin and those who are frequently in the sun should be advised to use sun screen.

EXAM TIP
Pearly, shiny lesion = basal cell carcinoma.

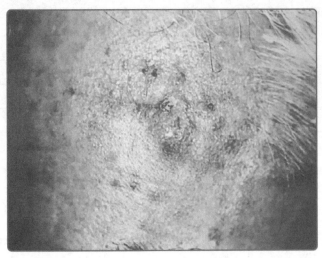

FIGURE 15-12 Squamous cell cancer is diagnosed by biopsy and removed. Reproduced with permission from Goldsmith LA, Katz SI, Gilchrest BA, et al: *Fitzpatrick's Dermatology in General Medicine*, 8th ed. New York, NY: McGraw-Hill; 2012.

Referral
- A referral to dermatology should be made if a suspicious lesion is noted.

BC. Malignant Melanoma
- Malignant melanoma is the most dangerous type of skin cancer (Figure 15-13).
- Malignant melanoma forms in the melanocytes (the skin's pigmentation cells).
- Remember the mnemonic ABCDE for the signs of malignant melanoma in a mole (Table 15-2).
- Watch for changes in the elevation of the lesion, firmness, and growth of the lesion.

Diagnosis
- Diagnosis is based on the biopsy of a suspected lesion.

CLINICAL TIP
Sunscreen goes a long way to prevent skin cancers.

EXAM TIP
A nonhealing or frequently bleeding ulcer should be considered suspicious.

CLINICAL TIP
A common site of malignant melanoma in women is the legs. For men, it is the back.

CLINICAL TIP
Caucasians are at an increased risk of malignant melanoma.

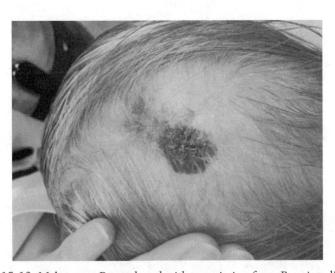

FIGURE 15-13 Melanoma. Reproduced with permission from Brunicardi F, Andersen DK, Billiar TR, et al: *Schwartz's Principles of Surgery*, 10th ed. New York, NY: McGraw-Hill; 2014.

TABLE 15-2	The ABCDE of Malignant Melanoma
Asymmetry	
Borders (irregular)	
Color (dark, changes in color)	
Diameter (> 6 mm is concerning)	
Evolving (any change in the mole or any new symptom, such as bleeding or itching, is a warning sign)	

Treatment

- Treatment involves the surgical removal of the lesion and is more effective if caught early.
- Once the lesion has spread, further treatments may be required, and the risk of more serious injury or death is higher.
- Many individuals with melanoma have specific gene mutations; for example, BRAF and MEK.
  - Inhibitors of the BRAF mutation can be used very effectively in treatment; these include vemurafenib and dabrafenib.
  - One MEK inhibitor is trametinib.
  - Testing and treating for specific gene mutations allows an element of individualization never possible before in chemotherapeutics.

Referral

- Suspected cases of malignant melanoma should be referred to dermatology and oncology.
- If there are concerns of metastasized disease, a hematology/oncology consultation and systemic chemotherapy are indicated.

CLINICAL TIP
Malignant melanoma is less common, but more dangerous, than other skin cancers. It is also the quickest growing form of skin cancer.

EXAM TIP
Look for a question involving a rapid change in the growth or characteristics of a lesion.

16
Mental Health

A. ANXIETY AND PANIC

- Anxiety is a state of unrest in which nervousness, panic, and other emotions occur.
- There are many sources of anxiety, some of which are obvious (eg, school, work, financial, and marital stressors); in other cases, there is no obvious source.
- The signs and symptoms of anxiety may be difficult to notice (Table 16-1).

Diagnosis

- Anxiety is diagnosed based purely on history.
- The nurse practitioner needs to be a good listener to pick up on clues offered by the patient.
- In most cases, complaints are vague and will require follow-up questioning by the nurse practitioner.

Treatment

- Both pharmacologic (Table 16-2) and nonpharmacologic treatments are available for anxiety.

CLINICAL TIP
Anxiety can also be a presenting symptom of almost any kind of physiologic disease.

CLINICAL TIP
It is important to observe for behaviors that could be signs of suicidal or homicidal ideation or planning.

TABLE 16-1	Signs and Symptoms of Anxiety
EMOTIONAL/PSYCHOLOGICAL	PHYSICAL
Withdrawal from situations	Myalgia
Irrational fears	Shortness of breath
Anger	Fatigue
Depression	Chest pain
Emotional lability	Nausea
Violent outbursts	Headaches

TABLE 16-2 | **Anxiety Medications**

CLASS	NAMES	SIDE EFFECTS	MEDICATION INTERACTIONS
Selective serotonin reuptake inhibitor (SSRI)	Citalopram, escitalopram, fluoxetine, fluvoxamine, paroxetine, sertraline	Sexual dysfunction Worsening depression Weight gain or loss Change in sleep habits	Illicit drugs Tramadol Other psychiatric medications
Serotonin-norepinephrine reuptake inhibitor (SNRI)	Desvenlafaxine, duloxetine, sibutramine, venlafaxine	Sexual dysfunction Worsening depression Weight gain or loss Change in sleep habits Change in blood pressure Headache Fatigue	Illicit drugs Tramadol Other psychiatric medications
Tricyclic antidepressant (TCA)	Amitriptyline, doxepin, nortriptyline	Cardiac dysrhythmia Sleep changes Blurry vision Gastrointestinal (GI) disturbances	Illicit drugs Tramadol Other psychiatric medications
Monoamine oxidase inhibitor (MAOI)	Phenelzine, selegiline, tranylcypromine	Mania Seizure Serotonin syndrome Change in blood pressure Headache Sleep disorders Tremors Sexual dysfunction	Illicit drugs Tramadol Other psychiatric medications Cold medications Alcohol

CLINICAL TIP

Depression can also be a symptom of many chronic diseases.

B. DEPRESSION

- Depression is a mental illness characterized by a persistent lack of pleasure in activities and low self-esteem.
- Depression can negatively affect family life, work, school, sleep, eating, and overall health.
- Physical symptoms are sometimes present.
- Depression is usually of unknown etiology; in some cases, it may be related to drug use.
- Serotonin plays a role in depression.

Diagnosis

- Diagnosis is based on a history of low mood, lack of pleasure in activities, insomnia or hypersomnia, and change in sex drive.

Treatment

- Pharmacologic treatment involves medication such as SSRIs, TCAs, and MAOIs.
- Nonpharmacologic treatment options include cognitive behavioral therapy (CBT), psychotherapy, and family therapy.
- Severe depression may be treated with electroconvulsive therapy, a procedure done under general anesthesia in which small electric currents are passed through the patient's brain causing changes in brain chemistry.

Referral

CLINICAL AND EXAM TIP

Observe for suicidal or homicidal ideation.

- Psychotherapy is an important part of the treatment plan for patients with depression.
- Referral to psychiatry, psychology, or therapy with a social worker is warranted.

C. SUBSTANCE ABUSE

- Substance abuse is a psychiatric disorder in which an individual consumes a substance for the reason of altering his or her consciousness.
- Legal substances can be abused when they are taken incorrectly for the purpose of altering consciousness.

Commonly Abused Substances

Common prescription drugs that are abused include the following:

- Acetaminophen/oxycodone
- Alprazolam
- Diazepam
- Zolpidem

  Common illicit substances that are abused include the following:

- Marijuana
- Ecstasy
- Cocaine
- Heroin

  Common household items that are abused include the following:

- Aerosols
- Gasoline and solvents

Signs and Symptoms

- Signs and symptoms of substance abuse are often difficult to discern as patients often try to hide them from others.
- Common signs and symptoms are listed in Table 16-3.

Diagnosis

- A diagnosis of substance abuse is very difficult to make.
- There are urine and serum drug tests available; however, different states have different laws with regard to the use of these tests.

Treatment

- To initiate treatment, patients must be willing to participate.
- Therapy, including both individual and group, is a mainstay of treatment.
- Medications may be used in certain circumstances for the treatment of addiction:
  - Methadone is used to treat heroin addiction.
  - Benzodiazepines are used to treat alcohol addiction.
- Support groups such as Alcoholics Anonymous (AA) and Narcotics Anonymous (NA) are very beneficial.

TABLE 16-3	Signs and Symptoms of Substance Abuse
Delusions	
Mania	
Panic	
Paranoia	
Agitation	
Sedation	
Depression	

CLINICAL TIP
Both illegal and legal substances can be abused.

CLINICAL TIP
"Drug misuse" is the term used by the Diagnostic and Statistical Manual of Mental Disorders (DSM) for the abuse of prescription drugs.

CLINICAL TIP
Patients usually do not seek treatment for substance abuse until they reach "rock bottom."

CLINICAL TIP
Treatment usually does not work unless the patient truly wants to stop using drugs.

CLINICAL TIP
Observe for behaviors that do not appear to be congruent with optimal care; for example, changing healthcare providers often or not caring for oneself adequately.

EXAM TIP
Questions will likely focus on identifying a potential substance abuse situation.
If the question is about caring for this type of patient, patient safety is key.

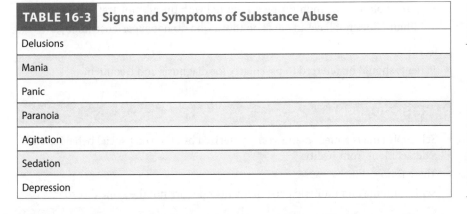

TABLE 16-4	Bipolar Disorder Presentation	
MANIA	**DEPRESSION**
Extremely elevated mood	Insomnia or hypersomnia
Decreased compulsion	Poor appetite
Lack of need for sleep	Suicidal ideation
Pressured speech	

D. BIPOLAR DISORDER

- Bipolar disorder is a psychiatric disorder in which the patient experiences violent mood swings, going from depression to mania in a very short period of time (Table 16-4).
- Patients with bipolar disorder must be screened for suicidal and homicidal ideation.
- Bipolar disorder is the mental illness most often associated with suicide.
- Symptoms of mania include grandiose thoughts, excessively high self-esteem, lack of sleep, flight of ideas, pressured speech (speaking rapidly), being easily distracted, engaging in highly goal-directed activity, and seeking pleasure.
- Bipolar 1 is characterized by the experience of at least one full manic episode.
  - A manic episode is a period during which the patient experiences symptoms of mania for most of the day for at least one week (or any length of time if hospitalization is required).
- Bipolar 2 is characterized by the experience of at least one major depressive episode and one hypomanic episode but no full manic episode.
  - In hypomania, the mood symptoms are not as severe as in full mania, and there are no psychotic features.

Diagnosis
- Diagnosis is based on clinical impression.
- The primary care provider must observe carefully for suicidal or homicidal ideation.

Treatment
- Psychotherapy is a must for the treatment of bipolar disorder.
- Medications for bipolar disorder are similar to those used in the treatment of anxiety.
- Treatment is dependent on whether the patient presents with mania or depression.
- Lithium is a common medication for bipolar disorder.
  - Careful blood level monitoring is required with the administration of lithium.
  - Lithium does not have an effect on those who do not experience mania.

Referral
- Patients should be referred to psychiatry for diagnosis and treatment.

E. SCHIZOPHRENIA

- Schizophrenia is a mental illness characterized by abnormal social behavior and a detachment from reality.
- There is no definitive cause.
- Schizophrenia and multiple personality disorder are not the same disorder.

CLINICAL TIP
Patients with bipolar disorder may present to their healthcare provider only when they are experiencing depression.

CLINICAL TIP
Patients may take their medication only when depressed, as they feel well during periods of mania.

EXAM TIP
Evaluating for suicidal and homicidal ideation is key.

CLINICAL TIP
Approximately 25% of patients with bipolar disorder contemplate or attempt suicide.

CLINICAL TIP
Flight of ideas, pressured speech, and grandiosity are characteristic of bipolar disorder.

- Age of onset is in the late teens to early twenties.
- Onset is often characterized by a psychotic break that may be violent.
- Symptoms include memory problems, cognition difficulties, disorganized thoughts and speech, and paranoia.
- Hallucinations are common in schizophrenia. These hallucinations can be auditory, visual, olfactory, or tactile.
- Substance abuse and alcoholism worsen the presentation of schizophrenia.

Diagnosis
- The diagnosis of schizophrenia is clinical; there is no definitive diagnostic test.

Treatment
- Treatment involves a combination of psychotherapy and medication.
- Medications include antidepressants and antipsychotics.

Referral
- Patients should be referred to psychiatry for diagnosis and treatment.

F. ANOREXIA AND BULIMIA

- Anorexia nervosa is a psychiatric disorder characterized by severe food intake restriction.
- Poor eating habits, an unrealistic body image, and fear of weight gain also characterize anorexia.
- Bulimia nervosa is a psychiatric disorder characterized by periods of binge eating coupled with purging (vomiting or taking a laxative to force diarrhea).
- Bulimia is also characterized by a distorted body-image and fear of weight gain.

Diagnosis
- The diagnosis of each disorder is based on careful history and physical exam (Table 16-5).
- The patient will likely show an aversion to gaining weight and have irrational dietary habits.

Treatment
- Treatment for both disorders is usually managed by a psychiatric professional with the primary care nurse practitioner monitoring the hemodynamic state of the patient.
- CBT, group therapy, dietary education, and lifestyle modifications are the mainstays of treatment for both disorders.

Referral
- Patients should be referred to psychiatry for diagnosis and treatment.

TABLE 16-5	Signs and Symptoms of Anorexia and Bulimia
ANOREXIA NERVOSA	**BULIMIA NERVOSA**
Obsession with dietary intake	Gastroesophageal reflux disorder (GERD)
Amenorrhea (late sign)	Dehydration
Abnormal dietary rituals	Esophagitis
Abnormal vital signs (late sign)	Constipation
Fatigue	Dental erosions
Dry skin and hair	Abnormal vital signs

CLINICAL TIP
Use caution when dealing with a person experiencing a hallucination; hallucinations are very real to those experiencing them.

CLINICAL TIP
Anorexia and bulimia may occur together or separately.

CLINICAL TIP
Anorexia and bulimia may be accompanied by comorbid conditions such as mood disorders, impulse control disorders, or substance abuse.

CLINICAL TIP
As a primary care nurse practitioner, your responsibility is not the long-term psychiatric care of patients with mental illness. Your role is to ensure that patients' vital signs and bloodwork are stable and then to refer them to the appropriate treatment provider.

EXAM TIP
For questions dealing with anorexia or bulimia, the correct answer is usually one that addresses the direct care of the patient, that is, ensuring they are not in immediate danger from electrolyte abnormalities, such as potassium deficiency, or at risk for suicidal behaviors.

TABLE 16-6	Signs and Symptoms of ADD and ADHD
ADD	**ADHD**
Lack of attention or focus	Easily distracted, lack of focus
Trouble keeping attention on simple tasks	Fidgeting
Not listening when spoken to	Constant motion, touching everything
Trouble following instructions	Difficulty performing quiet tasks
Easily distracted or forgetful	Trouble following instructions

G. ATTENTION DEFICIT DISORDER AND ATTENTION DEFICIT HYPERACTIVITY DISORDER

- Attention deficit disorder (ADD) and attention deficit hyperactivity disorder (ADHD) are disorders characterized by an inability to concentrate, with or without hyperactivity.

Diagnosis

- The signs and symptoms associated with a diagnosis of ADD or ADHD are presented in Table 16-6.

Treatment

- Treatment includes the use of medications such as amphetamine salts, methylphenidate, and atomoxetine.
- Psychotherapy and CBT may be used to develop focus and attention.

H. DYSTHYMIA

- Dysthymia is a mood disorder similar to depression but with less intense symptoms and a longer duration.
- Patients must be in a mildly depressed state for more than 2 years for this diagnosis.
- Signs and symptoms include fatigue, low energy, low self-esteem, appetite changes, and a lack of enjoyment in daily activities.

Diagnosis

- A diagnosis of dysthymia requires the following symptoms to be present for the majority of the time for 2 years:
  - Change in appetite
  - Change in sleep patterns
  - Lowered self-esteem
  - Fatigue
  - No episodes of mania
  - No episodes of psychosis
- Symptoms of dysthymia do not disappear for more than 2 months at a time.
- Symptoms cause social problems for the patient.

Treatment

- Treatment consists of a combinations of therapy and medication.
- The medications used are similar to those used in the treatment of anxiety and depression.

CLINICAL TIP

Although ADD and ADHD are often considered diagnoses of childhood or adolescence, young adults may present with either disorder.

CLINICAL TIP

Patients may go undiagnosed because the symptoms are very minimal.

CLINICAL TIP

Observe for indications of suicidal or homicidal ideation.

CLINICAL AND EXAM TIP

- Dysthymia = milder symptoms + longer duration.
- Depression = more severe symptoms + shorter duration.

TABLE 16-7	Medications and Substances that Can Cause Serotonin Syndrome
SSRIs	
SNRIs	
MAOIs	
TCAs	
Fentanyl	
Oxycodone	
Triptans	
Antivirals	
Antipsychotics	
Ecstasy	
Nutmeg	

I. SEROTONIN SYNDROME AND NEUROLEPTIC MALIGNANT SYNDROME

- Serotonin syndrome is a potential side effect of the overuse, abuse, or misuse of medications that affect serotonin.
- Cognitive, autonomic, and somatic effects are all characteristic of serotonin syndrome.
- Many medications and substances, legal and illegal, can cause serotonin syndrome (Table 16-7).
- Neuroleptic malignant syndrome is an adverse febrile reaction to antipsychotic or neuroleptic medications. When an individual's temperature is markedly elevated, seizures or rhabdomyolysis can occur.
- Signs and symptoms of serotonin syndrome and neuroleptic malignant syndrome are given in Table 16-8.

CLINICAL TIP
Serotonin syndrome is the result of an elevation in serotonin levels.

CLINICAL TIP
Neuroleptic malignant syndrome is the result of a decrease in dopamine levels.

CLINICAL TIP
In cases of suspected serotonin syndrome or neuroleptic malignant syndrome, other causes of symptoms, such as encephalopathy or meningitis, must be ruled out.

TABLE 16-8	Signs and Symptoms of Serotonin Syndrome and Neuroleptic Malignant Syndrome	
SEROTONIN SYNDROME	**NEUROLEPTIC MALIGNANT SYNDROME**	
Tachycardia	Cramps	
Sweating	Tremors	
Pupil dilatation	Fever	
Tremors	Diaphoresis	
Hyperactive reflexes	Confusion	
	Lack of balance	
	Coma	
	Seizures	

Diagnosis

Serotonin Syndrome

- Serotonin syndrome is diagnosed via the Hunter serotonin toxicity criteria: The patient must have taken a potential causative agent and have at least one of the following signs or symptoms: muscle jerks, agitation, diaphoresis, eye twitch, tremor, or hyperpyrexia.

Neuroleptic Malignant Syndrome

- Creatine phosphokinase (CPK) will be elevated.
- The patient will be taking a causative medication or illicit substance.
- Temperature will be markedly elevated.

Treatment

- Patients require emergency department (ED) admission and hospitalization.
- In the ED, patients may receive activated charcoal to absorb recently ingested oral medications.
- Sedatives may be given for agitation or clonus.
- Medications to relieve muscle stiffness and reduce temperature are given if needed.
- Fluids are given if needed.
- No specific drug therapy reverses serotonin syndrome.
- Dantrolene or dopamine agonists, such as cabergoline, are given for neuroleptic malignant syndrome.

Referral

- Suspected cases of serotonin syndrome or neuroleptic malignant syndrome should be referred to the ED immediately.

J. POST-TRAUMATIC STRESS DISORDER

- Post-traumatic stress disorder (PTSD) is a mental disorder characterized by symptoms arising from a traumatic event such as war, rape, or a near-death experience.

Diagnosis

A diagnosis of PTSD is based on a history of a serious, traumatic event and symptoms lasting more than 1 month. Symptoms include the following:

- Hypervigilance
- Difficulty concentrating
- Exaggerated responses
- Symptoms of depression and/or anxiety
- Sleep disturbance

Treatment

- Treatment consists of psychotherapy (including CBT) and medications similar to those used in the treatment of anxiety and depression.

K. SLEEP DISORDERS

Causes of sleep disorders include the following:

- Anxiety
- Depression
- Physiologic sources (eg, major medical illnesses)
- Medication side effects

CLINICAL TIP
In serotonin syndrome and neuroleptic malignant syndrome, it is key to stop the causative medication.

CLINICAL AND EXAM TIP
Serotonin syndrome and neuroleptic malignant syndrome are serious emergent conditions that require immediate diagnosis and management in the emergency setting.

CLINICAL TIP
Any event that is considered by the patient to be traumatic can trigger PTSD.

CLINICAL TIP
Observe for substance abuse in this population.

EXAM TIP
A traumatic event is required for the diagnosis of PTSD.

Diagnosis

- Diagnosis is based on history.
- The patient will describe trouble falling asleep, staying asleep, or some combination of the two.
- A sleep study can be conducted to rule out sleep apnea (a temporary cessation of breathing while sleeping).
- In cases of insomnia, it is imperative to rule out organic sources.

Treatment

- Treatment for sleep disorders can be difficult.
- The following medications may be used:
  - Sedatives; eg, zolpidem, temazepam
  - Antidepressants; eg, amitriptyline, trazodone
  - Over-the-counter remedies; eg, diphenhydramine, melatonin

CLINICAL AND EXAM TIP
Make sure there is no physical source of insomnia before assuming it is psychiatric in origin.

CLINICAL TIP
Sleep disorders such as sleep apnea have been linked with stroke.

17

Head, Eyes, Ears, Nose, and Throat

A. SINUSITIS AND ALLERGIC RHINITIS

Case 1

A 35-year-old female presents for nasal congestion, watery discharge, and itchy nasal passages and throat. The patient denies fever and chills.

What is the most likely diagnosis?

A. Allergic rhinitis

B. Sinusitis

C. Upper respiratory infection

D. Streptococcal pharyngitis (strep throat)

Discussion

The correct answer is A. Allergic rhinitis is rhinitis (runny nose) and postnasal drip caused by an allergy. The mucous is watery and nonpurulent, and there are no signs or symptoms of infection (eg, fever, malaise, myalgia). Sinusitis, upper respiratory infection, and streptococcal pharyngitis all have infectious etiologies.

Types of Sinusitis

- Sinusitis is a viral, allergic, or bacterial inflammation of the paranasal sinus mucosa.
- Sinusitis can be acute or chronic (chronic being more than 3 months in duration).
- The maxillary sinuses are the most commonly affected.
- Viruses make up approximately 60-70% of all sinus infections.
- Allergy is a more frequent cause than bacteria.
- Bacterial infections are more often associated with severe sinus pain, discolored nasal discharge, and fever.

Common Bacteria in Sinusitis

- *Streptococcus pneumoniae*
- *Haemophilus influenzae*
- *Moraxella catarrhalis*

Diagnosis

- Diagnosis is based on history.
- Nasal congestion or pressure, nasal discharge, and headache are the most commonly reported signs and symptoms.

- Tooth pain is often experienced with sinusitis.
- Transillumination will be diminished when inflammation is present.
  - Transillumination involves a light source being pressed against the sinus to see if light can be transmitted through the skin covering the sinuses.
- A computerized tomography (CT) scan can be helpful in the identification of chronic inflammation or a foreign object but is generally not needed.
  - If a CT scan is performed, mucosal thickening is commonly found.
  - A CT scan will be performed if the diagnosis is unclear or if recurrent episodes suggest the possibility of cancer.

Treatment

- Treatment depends greatly on the perceived cause.
- Symptomatic control consists of decongestants (eg, oral, such as pseudoephedrine, or topical agents, such as oxymetazoline).
- If an allergic cause is suspected, the following may be used:
  - Histamine H1 receptor antagonists (H1 blockers); eg, diphenhydramine (observe for drowsiness), cetirizine, loratadine, fexofenadine.
  - Prescription H1 blockers; eg, levocetirizine
  - Topical steroids; eg, mometasone, fluticasone
    - Topical steroids are first-line therapy for allergic causes of sinusitis
- Viral sinusitis is treated symptomatically with over-the-counter (OTC) H1 blockers, decongestants, and topical steroids.
- For bacterial sinusitis, one of the following regimens is a good choice:
  - Amoxicillin/clavulanate: 875 mg po bid × 7-14 days
  - Clarithromycin XL: 1000 mg po qd × 10 days
  - Levofloxacin: 500 mg po qd × 7 days

Referral

- If the sinus congestion is not relieved with first-line therapies, referral to an ear, nose, and throat (ENT) specialist is appropriate.
- An ENT referral should be first line if an abscess or other significant problem is suspected.

CLINICAL TIP
In viral and allergic sinusitis, 80-90% of cases do not require antibiotics.

EXAM TIP
Conduct an assessment before performing any procedures or imaging.

B. TONSILLITIS AND PHARYNGITIS

- Tonsillitis is an inflammation of the tonsils (Figure 17-1).
- Pharyngitis is an inflammation of the oropharynx.
- Both tonsillitis and pharyngitis are most commonly caused by viral infection (Table 17-1); however bacterial sources (Table 17-2) and allergic sources (Table 17-3) cannot be excluded.
- Importantly, most cases of tonsillitis and pharyngitis are *not* caused by group A *Streptococcus* and therefore do *not* require antibiotics.

Diagnosis

- Exudate is usually present in bacterial infections.
- The diagnosis of streptococcal pharyngitis is extremely likely if 4 to 5 of these criteria are present:
  - Pain on swallowing
  - Palpable nodes in the neck
  - Exudate
  - Absence of cough (cough originates in the lungs, not the pharynx)
  - Absence of hoarseness (hoarseness originates in the larynx, not the pharynx)
- In-office rapid strep tests evaluate for group A *Streptococcus*.

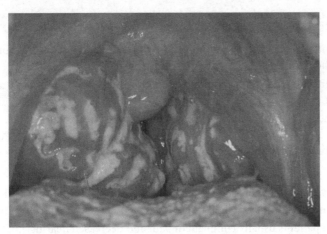

FIGURE 17-1 Notice the white exudate of bacterial pharyngitis. Streptococcus should scrape off when you press it, while diphtheria exudate will not. Reproduced with permission from Knoop KJ, Stack LB, Storrow AB: *The Atlas of Emergency Medicine*, 3rd ed. New York, NY: McGraw-Hill; 2010. Photo contributor: Lawrence B. Stack, MD.

TABLE 17-1	Common Viral Sources of Tonsillitis and Pharyngitis
Adenovirus	
Rhinovirus	
Herpangina/coxsackievirus	
Epstein–Barr virus	

TABLE 17-2	Common Bacterial Sources of Tonsillitis and Pharyngitis
Groups A and B *Streptococcus*	
Neisseria gonorrhoeae	
Mycoplasma pneumoniae	
Chlamydia trachomatis	

TABLE 17-3	Allergic Sources of Tonsillitis and Pharyngitis
Allergens that affect the respiratory tract; eg, pollen, cats, dogs	

- Throat culture and sensitivity are the most accurate diagnostic test.
- A culture should be done when the diagnosis is equivocal.

Treatment

- For bacterial pharyngitis, penicillin V potassium (penicillin VK) and amoxicillin are still the primary antibiotics used.
  - For penicillin-allergic patients, azithromycin or erythromycin is appropriate.
- Viral infections are treated with fluids, rest, hygiene, salt water gargles, and topical anesthetic sprays.

Referral

- An ENT referral should be made if chronic tonsillitis or pharyngitis is suspected.

CLINICAL TIP
Tonsillitis and pharyngitis are usually viral in origin.

CLINICAL TIP
For bacterial pharyngitis, penicillin VK or amoxicillin is the first-line antibiotic.

D. ACUTE OTITIS MEDIA AND ACUTE OTITIS EXTERNA

- Acute otitis media (AOM) is an infection inside of the tympanic membrane within the middle ear.
- Acute otitis externa (AOE) is an infection outside the tympanic membrane ("swimmer's ear").
- AOM and AOE present in all ages, but children are affected more often because of the anatomy of the Eustachian tubes in childhood (more horizontal versus the angle typical of adulthood).

Diagnosis

- A diagnosis of AOM is based on erythema, immobility or tautness of the membrane, and decreased light reflex.
- In AOM, patients usually complain of pain and decreased hearing.
- In AOE, pain, discharge, and itching are usually the primary complaints.
- Recent exposure of the ears to water is common in AOE because water changes the pH of the external auditory canal. Normal ear pH is low, which keeps bacterial growth down. Water raises the pH.

Treatment

- The best initial therapy for AOM remains amoxicillin.
- Augmentin, azithromycin, clarithromycin, or levofloxacin are the most commonly used antibiotics for AOM.
- Ciprofloxacin/dexamethasone otic or neomycin/polymyxin B sulfate/hydrocortisone otic are commonly used for AOE.
- Ciprofloxacin/dexamethasone is safe in perforated tympanic membrane.
- Antipyrine/benzocaine otic is beneficial for pain associated with either AOM or AOE.

Referral

- An ENT referral is indicated for recurrent or nonresolving AOM or AOE.

CLINICAL TIP
Observe for a perforated tympanic membrane. Perforation automatically requires an ENT referral.

E. GLAUCOMA

- Glaucoma is the increased pressure of the inner eye causing optic nerve damage.
- Testing is usually done by an eye specialist or a provider who is trained in tonometry.

Treatment

- Treatment is focused on decreasing the intraocular pressure or decreasing the volume of fluid in the eye.
- Constricting the pupil opens the canal of Schlemm and increases drainage of the aqueous humor.
- Medications used in the treatment of glaucoma are presented in Table 17-4.
- Laser therapy may also be used to create a drainage pathway.

CLINICAL TIP
Observe for acute angle-closure glaucoma.

Referral

- All glaucoma patients should be followed by an ophthalmologist.
- Patients should be referred to the emergency department (ED) for acute angle-closure glaucoma.

Emergency Situation

- Acute angle-closure glaucoma is an emergency situation.
- It involves a suddenly painful red eye in which the pupil is stuck at the midpoint.
- The eye will be hard and tender to palpation.
- The pupil will be nonreactive to light, and darkness may exacerbate the pain.

CLINICAL TIP
Caution must be taken with medications that can worsen glaucoma. This includes any medications that are anticholinergic in nature, such as tricyclic antidepressants (TCAs) and medications for chronic obstructive pulmonary disease (COPD), such as tiotropium and ipratropium. Acetylcholine constricts the pupil and opens the canal of Schlemm. Since acetylcholine constricts the pupil, any medication that has an effect like acetylcholine will be helpful.

TABLE 17-4	Glaucoma Medications	
CLASS	EFFECT	NAME
Prostaglandin analogue	Increases drainage	Bimatoprost, latanoprost, travoprost
Beta blocker	Constricts the pupil, opening the canal of Schlemm	Levobunolol, timolol
Carbonic anhydrase inhibitor	Decreases aqueous humor production	Acetazolamide, brinzolamide, dorzolamide
Alpha-2 agonist	Opens the canal of Schlemm	Apraclonidine, brimonidine
Miotic agent	Constricts the pupil, opening the canal of Schlemm	Pilocarpine

F. MACULAR DEGENERATION

- Macular degeneration is an eye disorder of the macula of the retina.
- Macular degeneration is the most common cause of blindness in elderly people.
- Macular degeneration results in central vision loss.
- Vision loss is bilateral.
- The external eye appearance remains normal.
- There are two types of macular degeneration: neovascular (wet) and atrophic (dry).
- Neovascular macular degeneration is more severe than atrophic; it develops rapidly, and the blindness is permanent.
- Diagnosis is by visual inspection of the maculaon dilated exam

Treatment

- An eye specialist should initiate treatment.
- Treatment includes vascular endothelial growth factor (VEGF) inhibitors, such as ranibizumab, bevacizumab, and aflibercept, which are injected directly into the vitreous chamber.
- VEGF inhibitors will either slow the progression of the degeneration or recover some vision.

Referral

- Patients should be referred to an eye specialist for treatment.

EXAM TIP
Macular degeneration is characterized by central vision loss.

G. RETINA PROBLEMS

- Many things can damage the retina; for example, chronic conditions such as diabetes, traumatic or atraumatic retinal detachment, and retinal artery or venous occlusion.
- Retinal pathology has origins in chronic conditions such as hypertension and diabetes.
- Acute conditions, such as detachment, occur as a result of trauma.
- Coagulopathy causes artery and venous occlusion, which is the sudden loss of vision in one eye.
- Retinal detachment is the sudden, painless loss of unilateral vision.

Screening

- Diabetic retinopathy should be screened yearly.

Treatment

- Treatment consists of photocoagulation.

- VEGF inhibitors are used to treat diabetic retinopathy.
- There is no clearly effective therapy for either arterial or venous occlusion. Anticoagulants are sometimes used, and in certain cases, surgical removal of the emboli causing arterial occlusion is performed, but no treatment has proved completely effective.
- For retinal detachment, an eye specialist will use surgery, laser surgery, or cryotherapy to place the retina back in its normal position.

Referral

- Any time a retinal condition is suspected, an immediate referral to an eye specialist should be made.

H. CATARACTS

- A cataract is an opacification of the lens of the eye.
- Cataracts are a common cause of blindness.
- Cataracts can cause difficulty with color determination and discerning contrast, which can lead to problems driving or reading.
- There are many common associations with cataracts (Table 17-5).

Treatment

- Treatment consists of surgical removal of the opacified lens.
- There is no medical therapy for cataracts.

Referral

- Patients with cataracts should be monitored and treated by ophthalmology and optometry.

I. CONJUNCTIVITIS

- Conjunctivitis is an infection of the conjunctiva.
- Common causes are bacterial, viral, and allergic.
- Bacterial infections are usually unilateral; viral and allergic infections are usually bilateral.
- Bacterial infections usually present with thick, purulent discharge.
- Viral and allergic infections usually present with thin, watery discharge, prominent eye redness, and itching.

Diagnosis

- Diagnosis is based on assessment and physical exam.

Treatment

- Bacterial infections are treated with antibiotic eye drops. Gentamicin or erythromycin are first line unless the patient has a comorbid condition such as diabetes, is immunocompromised, or wears contact lenses.

EXAM TIP

Cataracts are characterized by a yellow or white discoloration of the lens.

CLINICAL TIP

Early referral to an eye specialist is key to preserving vision.

CLINICAL TIP

- Purulent discharge = bacterial conjunctivitis.
- Water discharge = viral or allergic conjunctivitis.

TABLE 17-5	Common Cataract Associations
Aging	
Genetics	
Trauma	
Radiation	
Smoking	
Excessive light exposure	

- Treatment for patients with comorbidities is quinolone eye drops.
- Allergic conjunctivitis is treated with antihistamine eye drops, such as olopatadine and ketotifen.

Referral

- Patients with resistant conjunctivitis or persistent conjunctivitis, with or without periorbital cellulitis, should be referred to an ophthalmologist.

J. PERIORBITAL CELLULITIS

- Periorbital cellulitis is an infection of the skin around the eye (Figure 17-2).
- The condition is the result of a bacterial infection, commonly *Staphylococcus aureus*.
- Periorbital cellulitis is essentially managed the same as cellulitis anywhere else on the body.
- Patients typically present with pain and erythema around the eye.
- When extending into the eye, the condition causes pain on extraocular movements (EOM).
- Restriction in eye movement and blurry vision may also occur.
- The condition becomes markedly more severe if it extends into the eyeball and nerve; once this happens, the condition is considered orbital cellulitis.
- Orbital cellulitis is often caused by a gram-negative organism, such as *Haemophilus*, spreading into the eye from the sinuses.
- Orbital cellulitis can cause blindness.
- A CT scan can be used to differentiate between periorbital and orbital cellulitis.

Treatment

- Simple periorbital cellulitis can be treated with the same antibiotics used for cellulitis, such as oxacillin or cefazolin, or for methicillin-resistant *Staphylococcus aureus* (MRSA), such as ceftaroline, vancomycin, daptomycin, or linezolid.
- Later oral therapy is with amoxicillin/clavulanic acid or a cephalosporin, such as cephalexin, with close outpatient monitoring.
- Oral therapy that covers MRSA includes trimethoprim/sulfamethoxazole (TMP/SMX), doxycycline, and clindamycin.

CLINICAL TIP

When conjunctivitis is diagnosed, observe for periorbital cellulitis.

CLINICAL TIP

- Patients have a hard time remembering to put eye drops in, especially once they are feeling better.
- Patients tend to be more compliant with medications that require less frequent administration.

EXAM TIP

Always start with the most appropriate therapy (even if they are dosed every 2 hours).

EXAM TIP

Be alert for the type of discharge and whether the conjunctivitis is unilateral or bilateral.

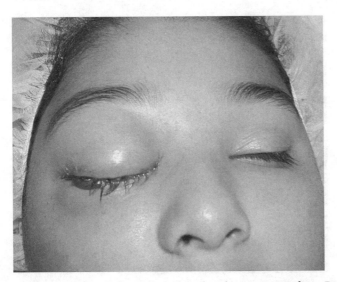

FIGURE 17-2 Periorbital Cellulitis. Reproduced with permission from Richard P. Usatine, MD and Usatine RP, Smith MA, Chumley HS, et al: *The Color Atlas of Family Medicine*, 2nd ed. New York, NY: McGraw-Hill; 2013. Photo contributor: Frank Miller, MD.

CLINICAL TIP

If orbital cellulitis is suspected, IV antibiotics must be started immediately.

CLINICAL TIP

In cases of periorbital and orbital cellulitis, always be observant for MRSA.

- Oral linezolid is reserved for the most severe MRSA infections.
- If orbital cellulitis is suspected, intravenous (IV) antibiotics must be started immediately.

Referral

- An eye specialist should be consulted whether or not the patient is admitted to hospital.

K. HORDEOLUM

Case 2

A 17-year-old female presents for swelling to the lower eyelid. The patient wears glasses but never wears contact lenses. There is no fever, no conjunctiva erythema, and no eye discharge. On exam, a white area on the inner lower eyelid is noticed. The nurse practitioner diagnoses hordeolum internum.

Which of the following is the common treatment for hordeolum internum?

A. Oral penicillin

B. Topical steroids

C. Topical erythromycin

D. Oral quinolones

Discussion

The correct answer is C. Topical erythromycin is the first-line therapy for hordeolum internum. Steroids are not indicated in this condition and are unsafe around the eye. Oral therapy is utilized when topical therapy fails.

Presentation

- A hordeolum (also called a stye) is an inflammation and infection of a sebaceous gland on the eyelid, commonly near an eyelash.
- A hordeolum can be internal or external.
  - A hordeolum on the inner aspect of the eyelid is called a hordeolum internum (Figure 17-3).
  - A hordeolum on the outside of the eyelid is called a hordeolum externum (Figure 17-4).

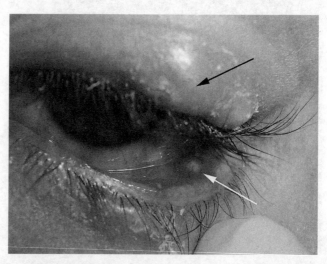

FIGURE 17-3 Hordeolum internum white arrive is internal hordeolum and black arrow is external hordeolum. Reproduced with permission from Richard P. Usatine, MD and Usatine RP, Smith MA, Chumley HS, et al: *The Color Atlas of Family Medicine*, 2nd ed. New York, NY: McGraw-Hill; 2013.

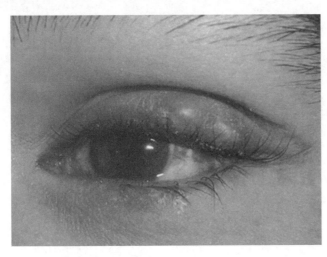

FIGURE 17-4 Hordeolum externum. Reproduced with permission from Richard P. Usatine, MD and Usatine RP, Smith MA, Chumley HS, et al: *The Color Atlas of Family Medicine*, 2nd ed. New York, NY: McGraw-Hill; 2013.

- The most common bacteria involved in hordeolum is *Staphylococcus aureus*.
- Patients typically present with swelling in a small, localized location.
- The affected area usually has a yellowish center and may have surrounding erythema.

Treatment
- Topical antibiotics, in eye drop or ointment form, are used.
- Ointments work better than eye drops as ointment tends to stay localized.
- Oral antibiotics may be considered if there is no resolution with topical therapy, if the erythema becomes more widespread, or if signs or symptoms of systemic infection develop (eg, fever).
- Warm compresses with a clean cloth are used to promote circulation and break up blockages in the infected duct.

Referral
- Hordeolum is usually well-treated by primary care.
- Ophthalmology may be considered if there is no resolution with treatment.
- An eye specialist should be consulted immediately if there is any change in EOM or vision in the affected eye.

CLINICAL TIP
Be sure to invert the patient's eyelid to fully assess the inner lid for hordeolum internum.

CLINICAL TIP
Patients with hordeolum may describe a scratching foreign body or irritating sensation when they open and close their eyes.

CLINICAL TIP
Quinolones are used if the patient is immunocompromised or wears contact lenses.

18

Musculoskeletal

A. SPRAINS, STRAINS, AND FRACTURES

Case 1

An 18-year-old female presents complaining of right wrist pain after a trip and fall. The patient is able to make all range-of-motion movements and denies point tenderness. However, there is pain with range of motion and mild bruising.

In this situation, which of the following is first-line therapy?

A. Wrist X-ray

B. Initiate a nonsteroidal anti-inflammatory drug (NSAID)

C. Emergency department (ED) referral

D. Orthopedic consultation

Discussion

The correct answer is B. As there is no point tenderness and the patient has full range of motion, fracture is unlikely. With a soft-tissue injury, NSAIDs and rest, ice, compression, and elevation (RICE) are first-line therapy. ED referral and orthopedic consultation are used for more severe injuries.

Presentation

- Sprains, strains, and fractures are typically the result of overuse or trauma. Occasionally they may be signs of abuse.

- Sprains and strains are usually graded on a scale of severity of 1 to 3, with 3 being the most severe.

- For patients, a good description of a sprain or strain is to think of what happens to a rubber band that is stretched over and over again: at a certain point, it will lose its elasticity (grade 1), and eventually it will not recoil at all (grade 3).

- Following repeated sprains or strains, rupture can occur. Rupture can also occur as a result of a sudden injury, such as when a soccer player with a planted foot is tackled.

- Most fractures are benign, that is, a result of trauma or repetitive motion (eg, stress fractures).

- The provider needs to be vigilant for pathologic fractures, which are fractures that occur as a result of malignancy.

Diagnosis

- The initial diagnosis of sprains and strains is clinical.
- Sprains will not show up on X-ray.
- Insurance companies will not pay for magnetic resonance imaging (MRI) during the initial phase of the injury.
- Following the joints through their normal range of motion is a good indication of the stability of structures.
- Joints should be assessed for laxity (looseness), crepitus (a grinding sound), or pain with range of motion or on palpation.
- Most insurance companies want to see a treatment of 4 weeks of NSAIDs and physical therapy (which can also be exercises prescribed by the primary care nurse practitioner) prior to authorizing an MRI.
- MRIs are very valuable as they can assess ligament, tendon, and minute bony structures much better than can computerized tomography (CT) scans or X-rays.
- If the patient has point tenderness, an X-ray is useful to rule out fractures.

Treatment

- Treatment depends largely on diagnosis.
- A good starting point is always RICE: rest, ice, compression, and elevation. This technique helps to prevent swelling and relieve pain naturally.
- An NSAID, muscle relaxant, or acetaminophen is a good starting point for pain management.
- Occasionally a narcotic pain medication, such as oxycodone/acetaminophen or hydrocodone/acetaminophen will be required.
- Physical therapy is beneficial in all strains and sprains.

Referral

- For all fractures, referral to an orthopedist is indicated.
- Depending on the primary care nurse practitioner's setting, an ED referral is also an option.
- Keep in mind that X-rays are required for the diagnosis and treatment of potential fractures, and splinting is often needed, but not all primary care settings are equipped to handle these tasks.

EXAM TIP

Always perform a physical exam before any radiology studies.

CLINICAL TIP

Because of the 4-week waiting period for an MRI required by most insurance companies, start NSAID and physical therapy as soon as possible (as long as it is safe to do so).

B. DIAGNOSTIC MUSCULOSKELETAL TESTS

Carpal Tunnel Syndrome Tests

- No blood test diagnoses carpal tunnel syndrome.
- Although an electromyogram (EMG) is the most accurate diagnostic test, it is generally not needed, and an MRI is definitely not indicated.
- An orthopedic referral and hand surgery are required following failure of a trial of NSAIDs.

Tinel's Sign

- Tinel's sign is a test for carpal tunnel syndrome that involves inverting the patient's wrist and tapping the inner wrist (Figure 18-1).
- Numbness, tingling, or pain is considered a positive result.

Phalen's Test

- Phalen's test is another test for carpal tunnel syndrome that assesses nerve impingement in the wrist bones.
- The test involves patient placing the backs of his or her hands together at a downward angle to the point at which the wrists touch (Figure 18-2).
- The test is considered positive when numbness or tingling occurs.

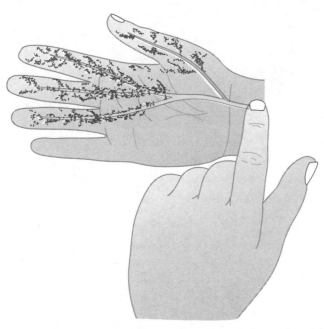

FIGURE 18-1 Tinel's sign. Discomfort reproduced by palpation of median nerve. Reproduced with permission from Sherman SC: *Simon's Emergency Orthopedics*, 7th ed. New York, NY: McGraw-Hill Inc; 2015.

The Finklestein Test

■ The Finklestein test is used to evaluate for tenosynovitis (an inflammation of the tendons in the wrist and forearm).

■ This test is completed by having the patient insert his or her thumb into a closed fist and pushing the fist downward.

■ A positive result indicates that tendonitis is likely and that NSAIDs and physical therapy should be initiated.

The McMurray Test

■ In the McMurray test, the patient lies flat with straight legs. The provider puts one hand on the patient's ankle and the other on the knee. The provider flexes the knee and moves the ankle internally and externally (Figure 18-3).

■ A click or popping sound is the sign of a positive test.

■ A positive test may indicate a meniscus abnormality.

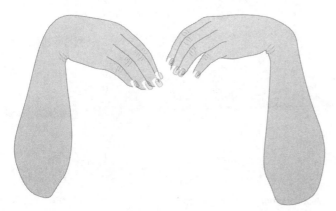

FIGURE 18-2 Phalen's sign reproduces the pain of carpal tunnel with compression by bending the hands. Reproduced with permission from American Society for Surgery of the Hand: *The Hand: Examination and Diagnosis*, 3rd ed. Philadelphia: Churchill Livingstone; 1990.

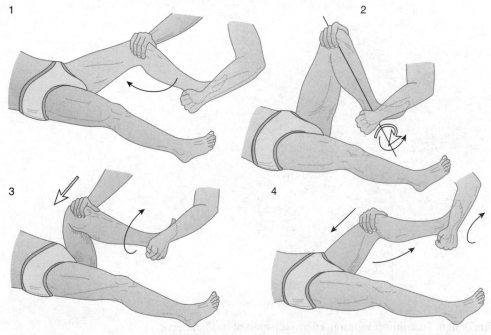

FIGURE 18-3 Mcmurray's test looking for meniscal tear. Reproduced with permission from *American Academy of Orthopaedic Surgeons: Athletic Training and Sports Medicine*, 2nd ed. Rosemont, IL: American Academy of Orthopaedic Surgeons, 1991.

CLINICAL TIP
RICE is always a good step to take with patients with musculoskeletal pains.

EXAM TIP
A physical exam is always preferred to imaging.

EXAM TIP
Know the names of the tests, how they are performed, and what they test for.

The Anterior Drawer Test

■ The anterior drawer test is a diagnostic knee test that assesses the stability of the anterior and posterior cruciate ligaments.

■ In the test, the provider stabilizes the patient's foot and pushes and pulls the knee anteriorly and posteriorly (Figure 18-4).

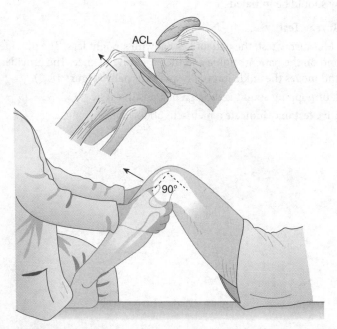

ACL: anterior cruciate ligament

FIGURE 18-4 Anterior drawer test assesses knee instability based on excess mobility from acl tear. Reproduced with permission from Imboden JB, Hellmann DB, Stone JH, et al: *CURRENT Diagnosis & Treatment: Rheumatology*, 3rd ed. New York, NY: McGraw-Hill; 2013.

C. OSTEOARTHRITIS AND RHEUMATOID ARTHRITIS

- Osteoarthritis (OA) is a degenerative form of arthritis caused by wear and tear on the joints. OA typically presents in midlife but can present earlier.
- Unlike OA, rheumatoid arthritis (RA) is an autoimmune condition in which the immune system attacks the body's joint spaces.
- OA tends to be unilateral, whereas RA tends to be bilateral.
- OA presents most commonly in the neck, low back (lumbar spine), fingers and toes, knees, and hips.
- RA presents most commonly in the proximal interphalangeal (PIP) joints of the hands and feet.
- OA typically involves a single joint in the lower body, such as a knee, hip, or ankle, whereas RA tends to affect multiple joints.

Diagnosis

- The diagnosis of OA is mostly clinical, but imaging, such as X-ray, may be helpful.
- If any other type of pathology is suspected, an MRI or CT scan can be helpful in diagnosis.
- There are no laboratory exams to diagnose OA.
- Blood tests in OA are normal by definition of the disease.
- A diagnosis of RA requires an abnormal blood test showing signs of inflammation (Table 18-1).
- In OA, there are no findings outside the joints.
- In RA, there may be comorbid findings, such as involvement of the lungs or coronary arteries, neuropathy, or anemia.

Treatment

Osteoarthritis

- The initial and primary treatment for OA should be acetaminophen; this is because of the adverse effects of NSAID use. (Chronic NSAID use leads to peptic ulcer in at least 10% of patients.)
- Other medications that may be used include tramadol, NSAIDs, and narcotic pain agents.
- Severe OA may be treated with hyaluronic acid injection at the painful site.
- Glucosamine and chondroitin are no more effective than placebo.

Rheumatoid Arthritis

- In RA, methotrexate should be used as a disease-modifying antirheumatic drug (DMARD) as soon as the diagnosis is made.
- About 40% of RA patients will need a second drug, such as a tumor necrosis factor (TNF) inhibitor (eg, adalimumab, etanercept, infliximab).
- A positive purified protein derivative (PPD) result must be excluded before initiating a TNF inhibitor.

TABLE 18-1	Diagnostic Blood Tests for Rheumatoid Arthritis
Antinuclear antibody (ANA)	
Erythrocyte sedimentation rate (ESR)	
C-reactive protein (CRP)	
Rheumatoid factor (RF)	
Anticyclic citrullinated peptide (anti-CCP) antibody: very specific for RA	

CLINICAL TIP

For patients on immune-modulating medications, careful preventive care, such as PPD tests, the flu vaccine, routine physicals, and routine bloodwork, must be instituted to prevent and monitor for infection.

Referral

- Patients with RA should be referred to rheumatology, as treatment may require medications to suppress the immune systems such as steroids, methotrexate, or other biologic agents.

D. GOUT

Case 2

A 60-year-old male presents complaining of persistent right great toe pain. He states that his diet has been heavy in meat and alcohol recently. The toe is red and tender to the touch. The patient is afebrile.

Which of the following should be the first-line treatment for this patient?

A. Febuxostat

B. Naproxen

C. Acetaminophen

D. Allopurinol

Discussion

The correct answer is B. Naproxen is an anti-inflammatory medication that works well for acute gout attacks. Hydration and a reduction in foods that provoke gout attacks are also beneficial. Febuxostat and allopurinol are not used in the acute setting but rather for gout prophylaxis following the acute attack. Acetaminophen is not indicated for acute gout.

Presentation

- Gout is a metabolic disease in which the body improperly processes uric acid. As a result, uric acid crystals get stuck in the joints.
- Gout commonly presents in the great toe, elbow, and knee.
- Gout tends to affect men more than women.
- Gout most commonly affects individuals in their 50s, 60s, and 70s.
- Patients typically present with one affected joint. (It is possible, but rare, to have multiple affected joints.)
- The affected joint will be red, swollen, and tender.

Diagnosis

- Laboratory tests will show a uric acid level > 7 mg/dL; however, note that uric acid levels may be normal during an acute attack.
- Needle aspiration of a gouty joint will show negatively birefringent uric acid crystals in the joint fluid.

Treatment

- Acute gout and chronic gout require different treatments.
- An acute attack of gout is addressed by reducing the inflammation. An NSAID is the clear first choice in this situation.
- If NSAIDs cannot be used because of ulcer disease or renal insufficiency, steroids are used.
  - Single joint involvement is treated by a steroid injection.
  - When multiple joints are involved, systemic oral or intravenous (IV) steroids are used.
- Colchicine is a third-line drug and not to be routinely used. Colchicine may cause diarrhea.
- Those not controlled with xanthine oxidase inhibitors, such as febuxostat or allopurinol, can be treated with a uricase medication.

CLINICAL TIP

The provider must be cautious in the approach to diagnosis to ensure the joint is not septic (infectious).

TABLE 18-2	Gout Diet	
DECREASE OR AVOID	INCREASE
Red meat	Complex carbohydrates
Poultry	Hydration
Fish	
Fat	
Alcohol	

- Pegloticase is a uricase medication used to break down uric acid in refractory gout. It is not used in an acute attack of gout.
- Chronic gout is treated with allopurinol or febuxostat.
- Dietary modifications must be stressed to all patients with gout (Table 18-2).

E. BACK PAIN

- Back pain is one of the most common causes for primary care visits.
- Musculoskeletal pain is the most common form of back pain.
- The most important issue for nurse practitioners is to distinguish the vast majority of patients who do not have serious pathology from the 1% who do and who may benefit from surgery.

Diagnosis

- A physical exam and history are extremely important in the diagnosis of back pain.
- Indications of the need for imaging such as X-ray or MRI include the following:
  - Focal neurological findings
  - Hyperreflexia
  - Extensor plantar reflex (upward response)
  - Bowel or bladder involvement
- An abnormal straight leg raise is *not* a sign of a focal neurological finding from cord compression or an indication of the need for an MRI of the spine.

Diagnostic Tests

- An X-ray will evaluate bony causes of pain.
- An MRI is the most specific diagnostic test; however, most insurance companies require a 4-week treatment of NSAIDs and physical therapy before authorizing an MRI.
- Certain situations require imaging before the 4-week time period often required by insurance companies (Table 18-3).

TABLE 18-3	Reasons for Early Imaging
Radiculopathy	
Possible metastatic disease	
Fever	
Hemodynamic instability	

TABLE 18-4	**NSAID Use in Back Pain**
NSAIDs must always be taken with food.	
NSAID contraindications include bleeding ulcers and renal disease.	

Treatment

- The first-line treatment for back pain is NSAIDs (Table 18-4).
- Muscle relaxants, such as cyclobenzaprine, carisoprodol, and tizanidine, may also be used.
- Narcotic agents may be used for intractable pain.
- Bed rest does not help.
- Fewer than 1 in 1000 individuals with chronic low back pain will benefit from surgery.

Referral

- Severe pain failing oral therapy may require an orthopedic or pain management referral for injection treatments.

CLINICAL TIP
NSAIDs are first-line therapy for back pain.

EXAM TIP
Always remember when an MRI is indicated.

F. LUPUS

- Systemic lupus erythematosus (SLE) is an autoimmune disease pathology of inflammation involving multiple body systems.
- SLE causes a vague range of symptoms including fatigue, joint pain, and rash.
- SLE can affect the brain, kidneys, bone marrow, and the body's cells.
- SLE affects females more than males.

Diagnosis

- Four of 11 criteria must be met to establish a diagnosis of SLE; however, only a few of these signs and symptoms lead to hospitalization.
- In joint pain, the X-ray and joint aspiration will be normal.

Systemic Lupus Erythematosus Diagnostic Criteria

Skin

- Malar ("butterfly") rash
- Oral and vaginal ulcers
- Discoid skin lesions
- Photosensitivity

Central Nervous System

- Confusion, disorientation, or stroke in young people

Hematologic

- Anemia, thrombocytopenia, neutropenia, or any combination of these

Renal

- Mild proteinuria, hematuria, or end-stage renal disease

Serositis

- Pleuritis or pericarditis

CLINICAL TIP
A malar ("butterfly") rash across the face is a sign of SLE.

Laboratory Testing

- A diagnosis of SLE is confirmed using the ANA test.
- ANA is 95%-99% sensitive for SLE but very nonspecific.
- An anti-double stranded DNA test is 60% sensitive for SLE but very specific.
- A positive anti-Ro test indicates a risk of neonatal lupus.

CLINICAL TIP
In SLE, anemia of chronic disease is more common than hemolysis.

TABLE 18-5	Systemic Lupus Erythematosus Medications
CLASS	NAME
NSAID	Ibuprofen, naproxen
Cyclooxygenase-2 (COX-2) inhibitor	Celecoxib, meloxicam
DMARD	Hydroxychloroquine, methotrexate
Opioid (used only in severe pain)	Acetaminophen/oxycodone, morphine, oxycodone
Steroid	Local injections for localized pain Oral therapy for systemic inflammation or pain

- Other common tests for patients with SLE signs and symptoms include ESR and a complete blood count (CBC).
- If anemia is found, it is most likely the anemia of chronic disease. Hemolysis with a positive Coombs test is also known aswarm IgG antibodies.

Treatment

- NSAIDs or steroidal anti-inflammatories are the cornerstone of SLE treatment (Table 18-5).

Referral

- If the ANA test is positive, a referral to rheumatology is warranted.
- SLE treatment is typically initiated and maintained by rheumatology.

19
Professional Issues

A. NURSE PRACTITIONER CERTIFICATIONS VERSUS LICENSURE

- The terminology of certification versus licensure is based on state policies. For example, in New Jersey, the Registered Nurse License is the primary license, and the Nurse Practitioner Certification is an addendum to that license.

B. COLLABORATIVE AGREEMENT

- Collaborative agreements vary state to state, and in a growing number of states, a collaborative agreement is no longer required.
- In states that do require collaborative agreements, the degree of collaboration required varies state to state.
- In most situations in which a collaborative agreement is required, the nurse practitioner retains the ability to function independently but must collaborate with their physician counterpart in certain situations.
- Facility Policy can override the terms of collaborative agreements.

Make sure you are aware of state, facility and practice policies as they may conflict.

CLINICAL TIP
It is very important that the nurse practitioner know all the rules and regulations regarding his or her licensure. The climate and dynamic of practice is ever changing, and new laws are regularly passed. Be diligent and stay current on what your state says you can and cannot perform in the course of your duties.

C. PATIENTS' RIGHTS

- Every patient over the age of 18 has the right to choose his or her therapeutic modality.
- The age of consent for minors varies for sexual issues, contraception, prenatal care, and substance abuse issues. The age of consent for these issues can be as young as 15.
- Once an individual has reached the age of consent, he or she may make decisions that the healthcare provider does not support and that could even prove harmful to the patient.
- It is not the role of a nurse practitioner to make decisions for his or her patients but to educate and inform them to the best of his or her ability.
- Personal feelings must be put aside and professionalism prioritized, even when healthcare providers disagree with a patient's decision.

D. CONSENT

- Consent is required for all manner of treatment except in the case of emergent, life-threatening conditions.
- Only adults may give consent (over the age of 18 in general, and over 15 for sexual health matters).
- Rules regarding the healthcare of patients under 18 varies by state; the most common to vary is the age required for an individual to consent to sexual health procedures (eg, birth control prescription or device implantation, abortion).
- For informed consent to be complete, the healthcare provider must provide full information about the benefits and risks of the recommended procedure or treatment.
- Patients have the right to rescind their consent at any time.

E. CHILD ABUSE, ELDER ABUSE, AND DOMESTIC VIOLENCE

- In most states, reporting child abuse is mandatory.
- In some states, healthcare providers may face legal repercussions for not reporting suspected cases of child abuse.
- Laws exist that protect the healthcare provider from prosecution if a report of suspected abuse ends up being unfounded.
- Elder abuse may be reported against the wishes of the patient, as the first concern is the patient's protection.
- Domestic violence should be screened for and assessed in cases in which the history does not fit the presentation, or if there seems to be an abnormal number of unexplained injuries.
- Domestic abuse cannot be reported against the patient's wishes.
- Situations such as suspicious burns or injuries and inconsistencies between injury and history should prompt the healthcare provider to be observant for potential abuse.
- Healthcare providers must not put themselves between the patient and the alleged abuser unless there is a direct threat.

F. LEGAL AND ETHICAL ISSUES IN END-OF-LIFE CARE

- End-of-life care is a legally and ethically complex area.
- Some patients at end of life want to fight until every possibly therapeutic option is exhausted, sometimes against your medical recommendations, whereas others will refuse treatments you may recommend.
- The opinions of family members regarding treatment options often come into play, as well.
- Treatment decisions at end of life are very personal decisions, sometimes based on religion or faith.
- An advanced directive is a legal documents stating the patient's wishes regarding healthcare in the event that he or she becomes unable to make those decisions.
- A power of attorney designates an individual to make decisions for a patient in the event that he or she becomes unable to make those decisions; the decisions must be in line with the patient's wishes.
- A do-not-resuscitate (DNR) order is an order written by a physician at the request of a patient. It instructs healthcare providers not to perform cardiopulmonary resuscitation (CPR) if the patient stops breathing or his or her heart stops beating.
- A do-not-intubate (DNI) order is an order written by a physician at the request of a patient. It instructs healthcare patients not to intubate a patient in the event of pulmonary failure. This order may be in place with or without a DNR order.

- A do-not-hospitalize (DNH) order is an order written by a physician at the request of a patient. It is used most often in the case of patients at end of life who do not want to be transferred to hospital for life-saving measures.
- There can be difficulty with these orders when family members do not understand them or try to override them. In such cases, the nurse practitioner must advise family members that such orders reflect the patient's wishes and are legal documents that must be followed.

Introduction to the Adult and Family Tests

Welcome to the testing section!

Here you will find questions similar to those you will see on the nurse practitioner board examinations, both the American Academy of Nurse Practitioners (AANP) and the American Nurses Credentialing Center (ANCC).

Adult/gerontology students, please use the adult test. Family nurse practitioner students, please use the adult test as well as the 30-question supplement of pediatric and OB/GYN content provided in the family test.

ABOUT THE EXAMS

- Remember: The material on the board exams is approximately 1-2 years old. In cases where information or practices have very recently been updated, you will not want to use the most up-to-date answer.
- There are 25 questions on the exam that do not count; these are used as evaluation questions for future tests.
- The exam includes content on complementary and alternative therapies. Do not discount an answer as incorrect simply because it is not a pharmaceutical answer.
- Remember your nursing process: Assessment always comes before diagnosis. Diagnosis always comes before treatment. On the exam, do not select a medication answer choice if there is also an assessment answer choice.
- The ANCC exam includes content regarding laws, regulations, and statutes. Make sure you are familiar with the most relevant ones.
- The AANP exam includes reference ranges for lab values.
- Both exams allow you to flag an answer and go back to it. If you get stuck on a question, flag it and move on.
- The exams are not designed to confuse you; the goal is simply to assess your basic knowledge.

TIPS AND STRATEGIES

- Get a good night's sleep the night before the exam.
- Don't overdo the caffeine.
- Eat properly.
- Remember to breathe!

Family Test

1. Which of the following types of fracture is suspicious for abuse?
   A. Compound
   B. Compression
   C. Dislocation
   D. Spiral

2. Which of the following types of abuse is mandatory to report?
   A. Spousal
   B. Child
   C. Adult
   D. Hate crimes

3. What pathology do Koplik's spots present with?
   A. Scarlet fever
   B. Measles
   C. Mumps
   D. Kawasaki disease

4. A 3-year-old in preschool presents with 4 days of fever (38.9-39.4°C), followed by a rash to the palms of the hands, soles of the feet, and throat. Which of the following is the most likely diagnosis?
   A. Kawasaki disease
   B. Coxsackievirus
   C. Mumps
   D. Measles

5. Which of the following is the best course of treatment for the patient described in question 4?
   A. Azithromycin
   B. Penicillin
   C. Supportive care
   D. Antiviral therapy

6. At what age is solid food usually started?
   A. 2 months
   B. 3 months
   C. 4 months
   D. When the child can hold his or her head up unassisted

7. A 30-year-old female who is 33 weeks' pregnant experiences some abdominal cramping, followed by severe abdominal pain and vaginal bleeding. Which of the following is the most likely diagnosis?

A. Placenta previa

B. Placental abruption

C. Labor

D. Miscarriage

8. What vaccines are recommended in pregnancy?

A. Influenza and Tdap

B. Influenza and MMR

C. MMR and hepatitis B

D. Tdap and MMR

9. Why is the measles, mumps, and rubella (MMR) vaccine not given until 1 year of age?

A. That is the age recommended by the Centers for Disease Control and Prevention (CDC).

B. That is the age deemed appropriate by the manufacturer of the vaccine.

C. It is a live vaccine, and the infant's immune system needs time to mature.

D. There are too many more important vaccines given prior to MMR.

10. Which of the following treatments is best for respiratory syncytial virus in a patient with mild respiratory distress and low-grade fever?

A. Supportive care

B. Azithromycin

C. Intramuscular ceftriaxone

D. Dexamethasone

11. Which of the following conditions can present with a red "strawberry" tongue?

A. Kawasaki disease and scarlet fever

B. Coxsackievirus and scarlet fever

C. Scarlet fever and measles

D. Kawasaki disease and coxsackievirus

12. How high should the fundus measure at 20 weeks of pregnancy?

A. The height of the symphysis pubis

B. The height of the umbilicus

C. None of these

D. Equal to the number of weeks in centimeters

13. Which of the following is considered advanced maternal age?

A. 30 years old

B. 35 years old

C. 45 years old

D. 40 years old

14. A 30-week pregnant female presents for a routine follow-up visit. Her vital signs are assessed as follows: blood pressure 140/90 mm Hg; heart rate 90 beats per minute; respiratory rate 18 breaths per minute. Her urine dipstick shows 2-3+ protein, and she has edema in her ankles and lower extremities. Which of the following is the most likely diagnosis?

A. Eclampsia

B. Pregnancy-induced hypertension

C. Pregnancy-induced proteinuria

D. Pre-eclampsia

15. When does pre-eclampsia become eclampsia?

A. When the blood pressure becomes uncontrolled

B. When a seizure occurs

C. At delivery

D. When the mother reaches 36 weeks' gestation

16. Which of the following types of burn is suspicious for abuse?

A. Burn from spilled liquid

B. Burn from spilled wax

C. Large surface-area burn

D. Multiple small circular burns

17. Which of the following medication classes is considered category D?

A. Penicillin

B. Sulfonylurea

C. Antihistamine

D. Angiotensin-converting enzyme (ACE) inhibitor

18. Which of the following medications is considered category X?

A. Penicillin

B. Trimethoprim/sulfamethoxazole

C. Methotrexate

D. Enalapril

19. Which is the following is *not* normal in pregnancy?

A. Increase in cardiac output

B. Decrease in peristalsis

C. Jaundice

D. Changes in skin pigmentation

20. Which of the following patients should receive RhoGAM?

A. Rh-negative mother with an Rh-positive fetus

B. Rh-positive mother with an Rh-positive fetus

C. Rh-negative mother with an Rh-negative fetus

D. Rh-positive mother with an Rh-negative fetus

21. At what age should a child be able to crawl or cruise?

A. 6 months

B. 8 months

C. 12 months

D. 9 months

22. Which of the following is a positive sign of pregnancy?

    A. Amenorrhea

    B. Nausea

    C. Fetal heart tones

    D. Breast tenderness

23. A 13-year-old female is brought to the office by her mother because she is always concerned about her weight. Her mother states that she is always reading the nutritional labels of foods. The patient's body mass index (BMI) is 15. Her vital signs are stable, and no complaints are offered. Which of the following is a possible diagnosis?

    A. Bulimia nervosa

    B. Obsessive compulsive disorder

    C. Anorexia nervosa

    D. Anxiety disorder

24. A 16-year-old female has yet to begin menstruation or sprout breast buds. The patient is very concerned about this. What should the nurse practitioner do?

    A. Reassure the patient

    B. Refer to endocrinology

    C. Perform a hormonal workup

    D. Initiate hormone therapy

25. A 3-year-old uncircumcised male complains of irritation to his penis. Upon examination, erythema is found on the glans penis when the foreskin is retracted. Which of the following is the most likely diagnosis?

    A. Phimosis

    B. Urinary tract infection

    C. Paraphimosis

    D. Balanitis

26. Which of the following is the best treatment for the diagnosis described in question 25?

    A. Nystatin/triamcinolone

    B. Oral penicillin

    C. Topical erythromycin

    D. Oral antifungal

27. When does ovulation occur?

    A. 28 days after the last menstruation

    B. 14 days after the last menstruation

    C. 20 days after the last menstruation

    D. 10 days after the last menstruation

28. The surge of which of the following hormones corresponds with ovulation?

    A. Luteinizing hormone

    B. Estradiol

    C. Follicle-stimulating hormone

    D. Progesterone

29. Which is the following is characteristic of Tanner stage 5 for females?

A. Breast buds, no pubic hair

B. Adult-shaped breasts and areolas, curly pubic hair

C. Flat chest, no pubic hair

D. Expanding chest, flat areolas, straight pubic hair

30. A 30-year-old female presents with suprapubic pain and vaginal bleeding for 2 days. There is suprapubic tenderness on exam, and the urine dipstick is normal. The abdominal exam is otherwise normal, and the patient denies nausea, vomiting, and diarrhea. An ultrasound is ordered, and a uterine fibroid is seen on the study. Which of the following medications is best for the pain associated with uterine fibroids?

A. Ibuprofen

B. Acetaminophen

C. Tramadol

D. Combination oxycodone/acetaminophen

Family Test Answers

1. D. Spiral

   Spiral fractures suggest physical abuse, since they are produced by a twisting motion, which is common in abuse. Compound and compression fractures are most often caused by trauma and are less often a result of abuse. Dislocations are not a form of fracture and not typically associated with abuse.

2. B. Child

   It is always mandatory to report suspected or known instances of child abuse. Reporting adult or spousal abuse requires the consent of the victim. It is not mandatory to report substance abuse as long as the individual is not putting others at risk. Child and elder abuse are reportable because they involve victims who do not have the ability to leave the circumstances of abuse. Remember that in elder abuse, it is not the age, but the vulnerability, of the individual that is relevant. Regardless of specific age, if an elderly person is unable to care for him or herself, and abuse is suspected or known, the abuse must be reported.

3. B. Measles

   Koplik's spots are a common presentation of measles. Scarlet fever presents with a textured, sandpaper-like rash. Mumps presents with a large mass in the neck. Kawasaki disease presents with a sunburn-like rash, bilateral conjunctival inflammation, "strawberrry" tongue, swollen lymph nodes, and high fever.

4. B. Coxsackievirus

   Coxsackievirus presents with high fever, followed by a rash. The rash is usually blister-like and is most common on the palms of the hands, soles of the feet, and throat. Coxsackievirus is the most common cause of hand, foot, and mouth disease.

5. C. Supportive care

   Supportive care is the only management recommended for coxsackievirus. Azithromycin and penicillin are not indicated, as this is a viral illness. There is no antiviral for coxsackievirus, measles, mumps, or rubella.

6. D. When the child can hold his or her head up unassisted

   While infants can usually hold their head up unassisted by about 4 months, some may not be able to until 5 or 6 months. In general, infants let their care-givers know they are ready for solid food by reaching out for it and taking it.

7. B. Placental abruption

   Placental abruption occurs when the placenta breaks away from the wall of the uterus. This produces severe pain and vaginal bleeding. Risk factors for placental abruption include car accidents, abdominal trauma, cocaine use, and hypertension. On the exam, one of these risk factors will likely be present in the question in order to differentiate placental abruption from labor. In the case of placental abruption, an ultrasound is done and will show a separation of the placenta from the uterus. Placenta previa occurs when the placenta is blocking (partially or fully) the internal cervical os. This typically occurs in the third trimester and results in *painless* vaginal bleeding. Miscarriage is not associated with pain and most often not with bleeding.

8. A. Influenza and Tdap

Influenza and Tdap vaccines are usually given during pregnancy. Since the influenza vaccine consists only of a viral antigen, there is no possibility of getting the flu from the flu vaccine. Pregnant women have a greater incidence of influenza complications. Tdap both prevents neonatal tetanus and provides herd immunity against pertussis. The influenza vaccine is given during flu season as applicable, and Tdap is given during the third trimester. Tdap is given in every pregnancy. The MMR vaccine is not indicated in pregnancy as it is a live vaccine. The MMR and varicella vaccines are considered dangerous in pregnancy. Although the hepatitis B vaccine is not dangerous in pregnancy, it is not specifically indicated. If the mother is hepatitis B surface antigen–positive, hepatitis B immune globulin and the hepatitis B vaccine are given to the baby immediately after delivery.

9. C. It is a live vaccine, and the infant's immune system needs time to mature.

An infant's immune system is not mature enough to receive a live vaccine, such as MMR, until 1 year of age. The immunity provided by vaccines is based on the reactivity of T cells, and T cells are not fully developed in newborns.

10. D. Dexamethasone

Since the question states that the patient is in mild respiratory distress, steroids to relieve the airway inflammation would benefit the patient. Supportive care is a good choice, but as the patient is in distress, it is not the best answer. In this case, supportive care would consist of hydration, acetaminophen, and antitussives. Antibiotics have no role in the treatment of respiratory syncytial virus.

11. A. Kawasaki disease and scarlet fever

"Strawberry" tongue can be present in both Kawasaki disease and scarlet fever.

12. B. The height of the umbilicus

At 20 weeks' gestation, the fundus (the top of the uterus) should be at the level of the umbilicus. After 20 weeks, the measurement from the symphysis pubis to the fundus should equal the number of weeks of gestation in centimeters.

13. B. 35 years old

Any mother over the age of 35 is considered to be of advanced maternal age and should be more closely monitored by an OB/GYN or nurse midwife than younger mothers. Amniocentesis may be considered by some mothers over age 35, as the incidence of many major genetic abnormalities, such as Down syndrome, increases after age 35.

14. D. Pre-eclampsia

Pre-eclampsia presents with elevated blood pressure, proteinuria, and bilateral lower extremity edema. Pregnancy-induced hypertension will not present with proteinuria or edema. Eclampsia presents with all the symptoms of pre-eclampsia, with the addition of seizures. Treatment of pre-eclampsia includes magnesium sulfate and blood pressure control. The definitive treatment for pre-eclampsia is to deliver the baby.

15. B. When a seizure occurs

Pre-eclampsia becomes eclampsia when the patient seizes. The treatment for eclampsia is to give magnesium sulfate and deliver the baby.

16. D. Multiple small circular burns

    While any burn can be the result of abuse, multiple small circular burns may be the result of cigarette burns. This presentation should be further evaluated for abuse. This type of burn is more commonly the result of abuse than the others.

17. D. Angiotensin-converting enzyme (ACE) inhibitor

    ACE inhibitors are considered category D medications. The other medications are considered category B. Antibiotics that are safe in pregnancy include the beta lactams (eg, penicillin, cephalosporins, carbapenems), erythromycin, azithromycin, nitrofurantoin, clindamycin, and metronidazole.

There are 5 categories indicating the potential of a medication to cause birth defects if used during pregnancy:

- Category A: Controlled studies show no risk or find no evidence of harm.
- Category B: Animal studies show no risks, but there are no controlled studies on pregnant women.
- Category C: Animal studies have shown risk to the fetus, there are no controlled studies in women, or studies in women an animals are not available.
- Category D: There is positive evidence of potential fetal risk, but the benefits from use in pregnant women may be acceptable despite the risk (ie, life-threatening condition to mother).
- Category X: Studies in animals or human beings have demonstrated fetal abnormalities, or there is evidence of fetal risk. The drug is contraindicated in women who are or may become pregnant.

Category C is the confusing category. A medication gets this classification if there is insufficient data on its use during pregnancy. It could be safe or probably safe, or it could be potentially harmful.[1]

18. C. Methotrexate

    Methotrexate is considered class X. While methotrexate is used for rheumatoid arthritis, it can also be used to induce abortion. The drugs for rheumatoid arthritis that are considered safe in pregnancy are sulfasalazine and hydroxychloroquine.

19. C. Jaundice

    Jaundice is abnormal during pregnancy; all other options listed are normal. Cardiac output increases by 50% because of an increase in plasma volume. The hypothalamic osmoreceptor alters in pregnancy so that the level of ADH is higher than in a nonpregnant person. This increases the amount of free water absorbed. An increase in progesterone causes a decrease in peristalsis and causes constipation. A change in skin pigmentation, called melasma, is also common in pregnancy.

20. A. Rh-negative mother with an Rh-positive fetus

    An Rh-negative mother with an Rh-positive fetus is the correct patient for RhoGAM administration. During the process of delivery, it is unavoidable that a small number of red blood cells should pass from the baby to the mother. If the baby is Rh positive, this leads to the development of antibodies in an Rh-negative mother. If the mother becomes pregnant again, the mother's anti-Rh antibodies will attack the Rh-positive red blood cells of the fetus, which leads to dangerous hemolysis in the fetus. This happens because the anti-Rh antibodies are immunoglobulin G (IgG), and IgG can pass through the placenta.

[1] Medication and Pregnancy. American Pregnancy Association website. http://americanpregnancy.org/medication/medication-and-pregnancy/. Accessed March 14, 2016.

21. D. 9 months

Babies should be able to crawl or cruise by around 9 months of age. Walking occurs around 12 months of age.

22. C. Fetal heart tones

Of the options given, fetal heart tones is the only positive sign of pregnancy. The other options are all presumptive signs of pregnancy.

23. C. Anorexia nervosa

Patients who suffer from anorexia nervosa are constantly concerned about their weight, always evaluate the nutritional content of the food they consume, and are underweight. Bulimia nervosa is categorized by binging and purging (by vomiting or laxative use). Patients with bulimia tend to have a normal weight and continue to menstruate normally. Patients with anorexia sometimes experience a decreased frequency, or cessation, of menstruation.

24. B. Refer to endocrinology

An endocrinology evaluation is recommended, as, by age 16, the patient should have begun puberty.

25. D. Balanitis

Balanitis is a fungal infection of the glans penis, which can be indicated by erythema of the glans. Phimosis and paraphimosis occur when the foreskin is stuck in one position, but in this case, the foreskin is able to be moved. Urinary tract infection would be suspected if the patient were having pain on urination.

26. A. Nystatin/triamcinolone

A topical antifungal is the best course of therapy for balanitis. An oral antifungal is not indicated at this point, and antibiotics are not indicated. Nystatin is a polyene antifungal that is chemically similar to amphotericin. Any topical antifungal, however, would be effective. Examples of topical azole antifungals are clotrimazole, miconazole, and ketoconazole. Another effective topical antifungal is terbinafine. Steroids such as triamcinolone are used to rapidly control the inflammation over a few hours.

27. B. 14 days after the last menstruation

Ovulation occurs on day 14 in individuals with a normal menstrual cycle. Fertilization happens within 24 hours after ovulation. The ovum should be in the distal third of the fallopian tube when conception is initiated with the sperm. Implantation happens by day 20. The trophoblast surrounding the fertilized ovum will develop enough to make beta human chorionic gonadotropin (beta HCG) by day 25. This is why a urine pregnancy test can be positive by day 25, before than the menstrual period would be expected.

28. A. Luteinizing hormone

Luteinizing hormone is the hormone that triggers ovulation. It is at its highest concentration during ovulation. Luteinizing hormone is also responsible for driving the production of progesterone from theca and granulosa cells after they have been turned into a corpus luteum. Estrogen is the primary sex hormone in females and is responsible for the development of all female secondary sex characteristics. Progesterone aids the menstrual cycle and helps sustain pregnancy. Progesterone maintains the secretions of the endometrial lining.

29. B. Adult-shaped breasts and areolas, curly pubic hair

The Tanner stages for females are as follows:

- Tanner stage 1: skin follows contour of chest, no pubic hair
- Tanner stage 2: breast buds form, faint pubic hair
- Tanner stage 3: breasts elevate off chest, pubic hair starts to curl

- Tanner stage 4: breast size increases, areolas form secondary mounds, pubic hair is curly but only on pubis
- Tanner stage 5: adult-shaped breasts and areolas, curly pubic hair

30. A. Ibuprofen

NSAIDs, such as ibuprofen, are the best pain medication for routine use in uterine fibroids. Narcotic pain medications should be reserved for severe pain. Patients with severe pain that cannot be controlled with NSAIDs should be referred for surgical fibroid removal via myomectomy or uterine artery embolization. Uterine artery embolization allows the removal of a fibroid by selectively shutting off the arterial supply to the fibroid through the use of a catheter.

Adult Test

INTRODUCTION

1. Which of the following medications should *not* be given with glucose-6-phosphate dehydrogenase (G6PD) deficiency?
   A. Trimethoprim/sulfamethoxazole
   B. Penicillin
   C. Nonsteroidal anti-inflammatory (NSAID)
   D. Morphine

2. A 24-year-old female presents for three day of fever, dysuria, and left flank pain. Which of the following diagnostic exams should be completed first?
   A. Urinalysis
   B. Magnetic resonance imaging (MRI)
   C. Complete blood count (CBC)
   D. The patient should immediately be admitted to hospital

3. Which of the following is the best location to auscultate murmurs of the mitral valve?
   A. Second intercostal space on the right sternal border
   B. None of these
   C. Third intercostal space on the left sternal border
   D. Fifth intercostal space on the left midclavicular line

4. After an unsuccessful trial of lifestyle modifications, which of the following is the first-line medication therapy for diabetes mellitus type 2?
   A. Metformin
   B. Glipizide
   C. Regular insulin
   D. Glyburide

5. A 35-year-old female reports feeling fatigued and that large amounts of hair are lost when she brushes her hair. She also feels cold all the time. Which of the following is the likely diagnosis?
   A. Hyperthyroidism
   B. Hypothyroidism
   C. Hypertension
   D. Hyperglycemia

6. For the patient described in question 5, what would you expect her TSH and T4 levels to be?

   A. Both TSH and T4 down

   B. Both TSH and T4 up

   C. Both TSH and T4 normal

   D. TSH up and T4 down

7. A 20-year-old female presents for sore throat, cervical lymphadenopathy, and low-grade fever. A rapid strep test is completed and is positive. Which of the following is the best initial therapy for this patient?

   A. Azithromycin

   B. Penicillin

   C. Moxifloxacin

   D. Clarithromycin

8. The patient described in question 7 returns to the office 3 days later with a rash. It is not pruritic, and the patient does not describe any signs or symptoms of allergic reaction. She does however state her fatigue is worse. A monospot test is completed and is positive for mononucleosis. Why did the rash occur?

   A. Rash is a known side effect of penicillin when used in mononucleosis.

   B. The rash is idiopathic.

   C. The rash is an allergic reaction.

   D. The rash signifies a life-threatening emergency.

9. Which of the following is the first-line therapy for isolated systolic hypertension in an elderly patient?

   A. Diltiazem

   B. Labetalol

   C. Amlodipine

   D. Metoprolol

10. What is the difference between a collaborative agreement and a supervisory agreement?

    A. A collaborative agreement requires electronic supervision at all times.

    B. A supervisory agreement requires electronic supervision at all times.

    C. A collaborative agreement requires direct supervision of all decision making.

    D. A supervisory agreement requires direct supervision of all decision making.

11. Which of the following screening exams needs to be completed prior to starting oral antifungal therapy for onychomycosis?

    A. CBC

    B. Liver function tests (LFTs)

    C. C-reactive protein (CRP)

    D. Erythrocyte sedimentation rate (ESR)

12. Which of the following is the antihypertensive of choice for patients with diabetes and no other contraindications?

    A. Beta blocker

    B. Calcium channel blocker

    C. Diuretic

    D. Angiotensin-converting enzyme (ACE) inhibitor or angiotensin receptor blocker (ARB)

13. A 24-year-old female presents complaining of sudden-onset fever, malaise, myalgia, and sore throat. Her vital signs are stable, and a rapid flu test is positive for influenza. Which of the following is the most common oral therapy for influenza?

    A. Azithromycin

    B. Penicillin

    C. Oseltamivir

    D. Fluids and acetaminophen

14. Which of the following medications should all ischemic stroke patients be on as long as there are no contraindications?

    A. Statin and acetylsalicylic acid (Aspirin)

    B. Metoprolol and aspirin

    C. Alteplase and statin

    D. Metoprolol and statin

15. A 65-year-old male presents for progressive tremor at rest, bradykinesia, and rigidity. The patient's daughter also mentions that the patient is not able to walk or stand with stability. What is the likely diagnosis?

    A. Parkinson's disease

    B. Myasthenia gravis

    C. Cerebral vascular accident

    D. Transient ischemic attack

16. Which portion of the neuron is destroyed in multiple sclerosis?

    A. Lewy body

    B. Myelin sheath

    C. The entire neuron

    D. Synapse

17. A 28-year-old female presents for 3 days of worsening left flank pain with minimal dysuria. She has a history of type 2 diabetes mellitus controlled on metformin. Her temperature is 38.9°C. Which of the following is a likely diagnosis?

    A. Urinary tract infection

    B. Gastroenteritis

    C. Pyelonephritis

    D. Colitis

18. Which of the following is the best outpatient antibiotic for the patient described in question 17?

    A. Trimethoprim/sulfamethoxazole

    B. Levofloxacin

    C. Cephalexin

    D. Nitrofurantoin

19. A 31-year-old male presents for muscle pain and fatigue. He reports that he has been exercising with great intensity and using protein shakes to train for an upcoming competition. The patient describes tea-colored urine. An in-office urine dipstick demonstrates hemoglobin. The lab urinalysis does not show red blood cells. Which of the following is the most likely diagnosis?

    A. Rhabdomyolysis

    B. Pyelonephritis

    C. Urinary tract infection

    D. Nephrolithiasis

20. Myasthenia gravis is the loss of which receptors?
    A. Norepinephrine
    B. Dopamine
    C. Acetylcholine
    D. Serotonin

21. When TSH is elevated in hypothyroidism, how should the dose of levothyroxine be changed?
    A. The dose should be increased.
    B. The dose should be decreased.
    C. Levothyroxine treatment should be discontinued.
    D. The dose should not be changed.

22. Based on the Eighth Joint National Committee (JNC 8) guidelines, which of the following is considered hypertension in an individual over 60 years of age?
    A. 120/80 mm Hg
    B. 130/90 mm Hg
    C. 150/90 mm Hg
    D. 150/100 mm Hg

23. Which of the following is the most common first-line antihypertensive medication for hypertension?
    A. Carvedilol
    B. Hydrochlorothiazide
    C. Diltiazem
    D. Labetalol

24. Which of the following is the most common site to hear a murmur associated with aortic stenosis, and what type of murmur is heard?
    A. Second intercostal space, right side; systolic murmur
    B. Fifth intercostal space, right side; systolic murmur
    C. Second intercostal space, right side; diastolic murmur
    D. Fifth intercostal space, right side; diastolic murmur

25. A 26-year-old female presents with diffuse abdominal cramping, nausea, vomiting, diarrhea, and blood in the stool. She denies fever and is able to tolerate fluids and a bland diet. Which of the following is the most likely diagnosis?
    A. Acute gastroenteritis
    B. Crohn's disease
    C. Cholecystitis
    D. Irritable bowel syndrome

26. If the patient described in question 25 developed fever, which of the following would be an appropriate next step?
    A. Initiate antibiotics
    B. Stool cultures
    C. Admit to hospital
    D. Initiate an antispasmodic medication

27. Upon physical assessment of a 70-year-old female with suspected diverticulitis, in which quadrant would you expect pain to be elicited?
    A. Right lower quadrant
    B. Right upper quadrant
    C. Left upper quadrant
    D. Left lower quadrant

28. Which of the following is part of routine management for a 50-year-old male?
    A. Digital rectal exam (DRE)
    B. Prostate-specific antigen (PSA) test
    C. Referral for colonoscopy
    D. Herpes zoster vaccine

29. Which of the following is a sign of hypokalemia?
    A. Dysuria
    B. Bloody stool
    C. Tachycardia
    D. Muscle cramps

30. Which of the following is *not* involved in the diagnosis of urinary tract infection?
    A. Leukocytes
    B. Nitrites
    C. Bacteria
    D. Ketones

31. On a bone density exam, which of the following T scores is indicative of osteopenia?
    A. Between 0 and −1.0
    B. A bone density exam is not a test for osteopenia
    C. −2.5 or less
    D. Between −1.0 and −2.5

32. An 18-year-old college student presents with 2 days of cough, congestion, and sore throat. There is no fever, and the exam is normal except for mild erythema of the nares and throat. The patient has not tried any over-the-counter medications. Which of the following is the most likely diagnosis?
    A. Viral upper respiratory infection
    B. Sinusitis
    C. Pneumonia
    D. Streptococcal pharyngitis

33. Which of the following is the best first-line treatment for the patient described in question 32?
    A. Combination decongestant/expectorant
    B. Azithromycin
    C. Penicillin
    D. Levofloxacin

34. The patient described in question 32 returns to the clinic 3 days later and now has a productive cough and a temperature of 38.3°C with rhonchi in the right base. The nurse practitioner diagnoses community-acquired pneumonia. Which of the following antibiotics would be an appropriate choice?
    A. Azithromycin
    B. Vancomycin
    C. Penicillin
    D. Doxycycline

35. A 30-year-old male presents with right lower quadrant pain and nausea that has progressively worsened over 24 hours. He has a temperature of 37.8°C. Upon examination of the abdomen, the patient experiences pain at McBurney's point. Where is McBurney's point located?

A. About halfway between the right iliac crest and the umbilicus

B. In the right upper quadrant, under the rib cage

C. In the left lower quadrant

D. In the right lower quadrant, near the pubic bone

36. Which of the following tests is used to evaluate for carpal tunnel syndrome?

A. Finklestein test

B. Phalen's test

C. Anterior drawer test

D. Tenderness at McBurney's point

37. A 30-year-old male complains of right elbow pain. No swelling is noted. Distal pulses, strength and sensation are intact. Which of the following should be used as first-line pain relief therapy?

A. Oxycodone

B. Ibuprofen

C. Nonpharmacologic therapy only

D. Acetaminophen

38. What is the term for a fluid-filled cyst that is visible under transillumination?

A. Hydrocele

B. Spermatocele

C. Epididymitis

D. Varicocele

39. A 25-year-old male presents with sudden-onset right testicular pain. Upon exam, there is a negative cremasteric reflex, and the right testis appears to be higher than the left. Which of the following is the most likely diagnosis?

A. Urinary tract infection

B. Epididymitis

C. Testicular cancer

D. Testicular torsion

40. Which of the following is the most appropriate course of action for the patient described in question 39?

A. Immediate emergency department referral

B. Outpatient testicular ultrasound

C. Urinalysis

D. Urology consultation

41. A 32-year-old male presents with low back pain radiating down both legs following a fall down multiple steps. The patient states that his buttocks feel numb and that he has been having trouble urinating. Which of the following is the most likely diagnosis?

A. Sciatica

B. Cauda equina syndrome

C. Lumbar radiculopathy

D. Spinal stenosis

42. A 42-year-old female with a history of anxiety presents for complaints of fever, myalgia, and tremors. She is on risperidone and tramadol. She recently had dental pain that caused her to go to the emergency department. The emergency department physician gave her tramadol for pain. On today's visit, the patient has dark urine and a temperature of 104°F. Her serum creatine phosphokinase (CPK) level is elevated. Which of the following is the most likely cause of her symptoms?

A. Parkinson's disease

B. Drug interaction

C. Neuroleptic malignant syndrome

D. Drug overdose

43. Which of the following psychiatric disorders is characterized by periods of depression offset by periods of hyperactivity and mania?

A. Bipolar disorder

B. Major depressive disorder

C. Anxiety

D. Psychosis

44. Which of the following is the leading cause of pelvic inflammatory disease?

A. Untreated chlamydia

B. Untreated gonorrhea

C. Untreated vaginal yeast infection

D. Untreated urinary tract infection

45. Which of the following is the most up-to-date treatment for uncomplicated chlamydia infections?

A. Azithromycin

B. Ceftriaxone

C. Penicillin

D. Ciprofloxacin

46. Which of the following is *not* an example of elder abuse or neglect?

A. Not providing appropriate clothing for the temperature

B. Hitting or striking an elderly person

C. Not providing medication or adequate resources

D. Providing support and time to adjust to new situations and surroundings

47. A 55-year-old male presents with left lower eyelid swelling and irritation. The patient denies conjunctival erythema or discharge. Upon eversion of the eyelid, a small, circular erythematous area with a central white spot is noted. Which of the following is the most likely diagnosis?

A. Hordeolum externum

B. Conjunctivitis

C. Chalazion

D. Hordeolum internum

48. Which of the following is the most appropriate evidence-based treatment for the diagnosis described in question 47?

A. Oral azithromycin

B. Topical erythromycin

C. Warm compresses with gentle massage

D. Oral levofloxacin

49. What is the red circular rash associated with Lyme disease called?
    A. Erythema migrans
    B. Rosacea
    C. Pustules
    D. Koplik spots

50. Which of the following is commonly the initial presenting symptom of human immunodeficiency virus (HIV)?
    A. Fever
    B. Blood in stool
    C. Hyperactivity
    D. Flu-like symptoms

51. At what point is human immunodeficiency virus (HIV) considered to have caused acquired immune deficiency syndrome (AIDS)?
    A. When the CD4 count is less than 150
    B. When the CD4 count is less than 250
    C. When the CD4 count is less than 200
    D. When the CD4 count is less than 50

52. A patient was diagnosed with bacterial conjunctivitis 2 days ago and started on tobramycin. The patient presents today with a complaint of fever and erythema around the left eye. The patient has full range of motion in the eye, and there is no change in vision. Which of the following diagnoses should the nurse practitioner be most concerned about?
    A. Hordeolum
    B. Periorbital cellulitis
    C. Conjunctivitis
    D. Chalazion

53. What would a complete blood count (CBC) look like for a patient with iron deficiency anemia?
    A. Low hemoglobin, low hematocrit, high mean corpuscular hemoglobin (MCH), high mean corpuscular volume (MCV)
    B. Normal hemoglobin, normal hematocrit, low MCH, low MCV
    C. Low hemoglobin, low hematocrit, low MCH, low MCV
    D. High hemoglobin, high hematocrit, low MCH, low MCV

54. What would a complete blood count (CBC) look like for a patient with B12 deficiency anemia?
    A. Low hemoglobin, low hematocrit, high MCH, high MCV
    B. Normal hemoglobin, normal hematocrit, low MCH, low MCV
    C. Low hemoglobin, low hematocrit, low MCH, low MCV
    D. High hemoglobin, high hematocrit, low MCH, low MCV

55. Which of the following describes the correct pathway of blood through the heart?
    A. Inferior vena cava, right atrium, tricuspid valve, right ventricle, pulmonary artery, lungs, pulmonary vein, left artery, mitral valve, left ventricle, aorta
    B. Superior vena cava, right atrium, mitral valve, right ventricle, pulmonary artery, lungs, pulmonary vein, left artery, tricuspid valve, left ventricle, aorta
    C. Inferior vena cava, right atrium, mitral valve, right ventricle, pulmonary artery, lungs, pulmonary vein, left artery, tricuspid valve, left ventricle, aorta
    D. Superior vena cava, right atrium, tricuspid valve, right ventricle, pulmonary vein, lungs, pulmonary artery, left artery, mitral valve, left ventricle, aorta

56. Which inferior leads of an electrocardiogram (EKC or ECG) would demonstrate ischemia or infarction?

A. Diffuse nonspecific elevations

B. II, III, AvF

C. I, AvL, V5, V6

D. V2-V4

57. Which of the following types of medication is *not* one of the mainstays for the treatment of congestive heart failure?

A. Angiotensin-converting enzyme (ACE) inhibitors

B. Calcium channel blockers

C. Beta blockers

D. Diuretics

58. Which of the following is *not* a defining feature of emphysema?

A. A partial pressure of oxygen (pO_2) of 60-80 mm Hg

B. Barrel chest

C. Edema

D. Dyspnea on exertion

59. A 28-year-old female patient presents complaining of a rash on her neck. The area is reddened with a honey-colored crusting. The nurse practitioner diagnoses impetigo. Which of the following is the most bacterial cause of impetigo?

A. *Streptococcus pyogenes*

B. *Escherichia coli*

C. *Staphylococcus aureus*

D. *Pseudomonas*

60. A 25-year-old female is being treated for mononucleosis. If the patient is suspected of having a concurrent throat infection, which of the following antibiotics should be avoided?

A. Levofloxacin

B. Doxycycline

C. Ampicillin

D. Azithromycin

61. Which of the following is the first-line blood pressure medication for a patient with diabetes mellitus?

A. Beta blocker

B. Angiotensin-converting enzyme (ACE) inhibitor

C. Calcium channel blocker

D. Thiazide diuretic

62. A 70-year-old male presents with left lower quadrant pain, nausea, vomiting, and bloody diarrhea. A computerized tomography (CT) scan demonstrates diverticulitis. After the patient is treated and released from hospital, which of the following dietary modifications should the nurse practitioner recommend?

A. High fiber

B. Low salt

C. Low vitamin K

D. No seeds

63. A 70-year-old female present complaining of right calf pain for 3 days. The patient denies numbness and tingling. The patient has recently returned from a trip visiting her grandchildren. Which of the following clinical tests for deep vein thrombosis can be performed in the office?

    A. McBurney's point

    B. Ankle-brachial index

    C. Anterior drawer test

    D. Homans' sign

64. A 75-year-old male has a long-standing history of hypertension and diabetes. He currently complains of right leg pain that worsens with walking. Which of the following tests for peripheral artery disease can be completed in the office?

    A. McBurney's point

    B. Ankle-brachial index

    C. Anterior drawer test

    D. Homans' sign

65. Which of the following medications for hyperthyroidism is best for a 34-year-old woman who is pregnant?

    A. Methimazole

    B. Propranolol

    C. Propylthiouracil

    D. Levothyroxine

66. Which of the following is a common cause of hypokalemia?

    A. Renal failure

    B. Crush injury

    C. Vomiting

    D. Combination spironolactone/enalapril

67. Which of the following causes hyperkalemia?

    A. Aldosterone-secreting tumor

    B. Black licorice

    C. Diuretics

    D. Diabetic ketoacidosis

68. A 24-year-old female presents for vaginal itchiness and thin, gray vaginal discharge. Which of the following is a likely diagnosis?

    A. Chlamydia

    B. Gonorrhea

    C. Yeast infection

    D. Trichomoniasis

69. A 34-year-old female presents for vaginal itchiness and thick, white, cottage cheese–like vaginal discharge. Which of the following is a likely diagnosis?

    A. Chlamydia

    B. Gonorrhea

    C. Yeast infection

    D. Trichomoniasis

70. A 40-year-old male presents for nausea, vomiting, diarrhea, and right upper quadrant pain. He recently returned from Mexico. His bloodwork is positive for hepatitis A immunoglobulin (IgM) and hepatitis B surface antibody and negative for hepatitis B IgM and hepatitis C IgM. Which of the following is the treatment for this patient?

  A. Intravenous immunoglobulin

  B. Intravenous antibiotics

  C. Supportive care

  D. Oral antivirals

71. What is the mnemonic used to evaluate for substance abuse?

  A. CAGE

  B. OPQRST

  C. OLDCARTS

  D. ABC

72. An 18-year-old male presents complaining of more than 6 months of diffuse abdominal cramping and bloating that culminates in diarrhea. There is no nausea, vomiting, fever, or chills. The patient states that the bloating, pain, and diarrhea seem to be correlated with anxiety. There is no blood or mucous in the stool. Which of the following is the most likely diagnosis?

  A. Irritable bowel syndrome

  B. Crohn's disease

  C. Gastroenteritis

  D. Ulcerative colitis

73. Which of the following is a common genetic abnormality seen in breast cancer?

  A. Lynch syndrome

  B. Li-Fraumeni syndrome

  C. BRCA1 and BRCA2 gene mutations

  D. Cowden syndrome

74. A 18-year-old male presents complaining of right testicular pain starting 1 hour prior to arrival. The nurse practitioner suspects torsion. Which of the following assessment reflexes should be elicited?

  A. Cremasteric reflex

  B. Urinalysis

  C. Blue dot sign

  D. Murphy's sign

75. A patient with suspected ovarian torsion has approximately how long for proper assessment, diagnosis, and treatment prior to the death of the ovary?

  A. 10 hours

  B. 12 hours

  C. 6 hours

  D. 24 hours

76. Which of the following is the cause of symptoms in relapsing-remitting multiple sclerosis?

  A. The presence of Lewy bodies

  B. Demyelination of the neurons

  C. Destruction of the hypothalamus

  D. Inflammation of the meninges

77. Which of the following is the characteristic tremor of Parkinson's disease?
    A. Tremor with movement
    B. Tremor with stress
    C. No tremor is noted in Parkinson's disease.
    D. Resting tremor

78. Which cranial nerve is affected in Bell's palsy?
    A. V
    B. III
    C. VII
    D. X

79. Which of the following is the most common cause of intertrigo in obese female patients with diabetes?
    A. *Streptococcus*
    B. *Candida*
    C. *Pseudomonas*
    D. *Staphylococcus*

80. Which of the following is the first-line treatment for intertrigo?
    A. Oral antibiotic
    B. Oral antifungal
    C. Topical antibiotic
    D. Topical antifungal

81. If terbinafine is to be initiated, which of the followings baseline laboratory evaluations should be ordered?
    A. Complete blood count
    B. Basic metabolic profile
    C. Liver function tests (LFTs)
    D. Hepatitis panel

82. A 25-year-old male patient with eczema and asthma asks why every time one condition flares up, so does the other. What is the best response the nurse practitioner can give?
    A. It is a coincidence.
    B. The reason for this is unknown.
    C. Both conditions are caused by bacteria; the patient should be advised to wash his hands more often.
    D. Both conditions have allergic triggers.

83. An 80-year-old female presents with multiple small growths on her neck and shoulders. The lesions are not scaly, erythematous, or painful, and they have not changed in size recently. Which of the following is a likely diagnosis?
    A. Basal cell carcinoma
    B. Squamous cell carcinoma
    C. Acne
    D. Seborrheic dermatitis

84. Macular degeneration results in a loss of which of the following?
    A. Central vision
    B. Peripheral vision
    C. All vision
    D. Color vision

85. A 75-year-old male presents with severe right eye pain and vision loss starting approximately 30 minutes ago. The nurse practitioner diagnoses acute angle-closure glaucoma. Which of the following is the best course of action?

    A. Contact an ophthalmologist

    B. Refer to the emergency department

    C. Initiate an oral beta blocker

    D. Initiate a topical antibiotic

86. Which of the following is a complementary and alternative medicine (CAM) for sinusitis?

    A. Steroid nasal spray

    B. Massage therapy

    C. Nasal irrigation with distilled water

    D. Yoga

87. Which of the following is *not* a potential cause of temporomandibular joint (TMJ) disorder?

    A. Stress

    B. Chewing gum

    C. Bruxism

    D. Talking

88. Which of the following *is not* an examination for tuberculosis?

    A. Chest X-ray

    B. Purified protein derivative (PPD)

    C. QuantiFERON-TB Gold (QFT-G)

    D. Isoniazid

89. What is a fundamental difference between asthma and chronic obstructive pulmonary disease (COPD)?

    A. Asthma is reversible.

    B. COPD is reversible.

    C. Neither is reversible.

    D. Reversibility is not a characteristic of either asthma or COPD.

90. Which of the following statements regarding asthma is *not* correct?

    A. Mild intermittent asthma requires no daily medications.

    B. Mild persistent asthma may require the use of a daily inhaled steroid.

    C. Moderate persistent asthma may require the use of a daily inhaled steroid and long-acting beta agonist.

    D. Severe persistent asthma requires intubation.

91. Which of the following is true regarding the forced expiratory volume during the first second of the forced breath (FEV1) in a pulmonary function test (PFT)?

    A. 60-80% is normal.

    B. Below 80% is normal.

    C. 70-90% is normal.

    D. Below 80% is abnormal.

92. What does an FEV1 below 80% indicate?
    A. Obstruction
    B. A poorly performed test
    C. Wheezing
    D. Normal lung function

93. Which of the following contributes most to a patient's success in quitting smoking?
    A. The patient's insurance company covers the cost of the medication.
    B. The patient actively wants to quit smoking.
    C. The patient's family wants the patient to quit smoking.
    D. The patient has several smoking-related comorbidities.

94. Which of the following is a common side effect of varenicline treatment?
    A. Suicidality
    B. Vivid dreams
    C. Nausea
    D. Sleepwalking

95. A nurse practitioner is doing an exam on an 85-year-old male with abdominal pain. The past medical history is significant for smoking, hypertension, diabetes, and dyslipidemia. Upon palpation of the abdomen, the nurse practitioner feels a pulsatile mass. Which of the following is the best course of treatment?
    A. Call 911
    B. Vascular surgery
    C. Outpatient CT scan
    D. Strict blood pressure control

96. Which of the following is the definition of metabolic syndrome?
    A. Elevated body mass index (BMI), normal systolic blood pressure (SBP), elevated triglycerides, elevated glucose, normal high-density lipoprotein (HDL)
    B. Elevated BMI, elevated SBP, elevated triglycerides, decreased glucose, elevated HDL
    C. Elevated BMI, elevated SBP, elevated triglycerides, elevated glucose, decreased HDL
    D. Elevated BMI, decreased SBP, elevated triglycerides, elevated glucose, decreased HDL

97. How many grades of cardiac murmur exist?
    A. 10
    B. 4
    C. 6
    D. 3

98. At what stage can a cardiac murmur be auscultated with a regular stethoscope?
    A. 1
    B. 2-3
    C. 4-5
    D. 6

99. How is the murmur associated with mitral valve prolapse described?

    A. Late-systolic click

    B. Early-systolic blowing

    C. Early-diastolic blowing

    D. Late-diastolic click

100. Which of the following is *not* a risk factor for deep vein thrombosis?

    A. Sedentary lifestyle

    B. Pregnancy

    C. Admission to hospital for observation

    D. Trauma or surgery

101. Which of the following is a normal side effect of pink bismuth?

    A. Dark stool

    B. Red stool

    C. Fever

    D. Right lower quadrant pain

102. A patient with pheochromocytoma presents for preoperative clearance prior to the tumor being removed. What must be completed prior to surgery?

    A. Strict blood pressure control

    B. Endocrinology consultation

    C. Glucose control

    D. None of the above

103. Why is cranberry extract used as a complementary and alternative medicine (CAM) for urinary tract infection?

    A. For its anesthetic properties

    B. For its bactericidal properties

    C. To decrease bacterial reproduction

    D. To decrease the adherence of bacteria to tissue

104. Which of the following is *not* a cause of erectile dysfunction?

    A. Stress

    B. Benign prostatic hyperplasia (BPH)

    C. Diuretics

    D. Diabetes

105. A 60-year-old male patient presents with complaints of rectal pain, dysuria, and fever. There is no nausea, vomiting, or diarrhea. Which of the following is a likely diagnosis?

    A. Urinary tract infection

    B. Prostatitis

    C. Colitis

    D. Pyelonephritis

106. Which of the following is *not* a common bacterium involved in the diagnosis described in in question 105?

    A. *Escherichia coli*

    B. *Klebsiella pseudomonas*

    C. *Streptococcus pneumoniae*

    D. *Proteus*

107. Which of the following is the second most common cancer in the United States?
    A. Lung
    B. Breast
    C. Prostate
    D. Colon

108. What is the reference range for potassium?
    A. 3.5-5.0 mEq/L
    B. 135-145 mEq/L
    C. 10-20 mEq/L
    D. 8-10 mEq/L

109. What is the reference range for sodium?
    A. 3.5-5.0 mEq/L
    B. 135-145 mEq/L
    C. 10-20 mEq/L
    D. 8-10 mEq/L

110. A patient presents for right great toe redness, swelling, and pain. A STAT uric acid level is drawn and comes back with a reading of 9.2 mg/dL. Which of the following is an appropriate first-line treatment?
    A. Colchicine
    B. Ibuprofen
    C. Allopurinol
    D. Febuxostat

111. Which of the following is *not* a common cause of dyspareunia?
    A. Sexually transmitted disease
    B. Urinary tract infection
    C. None of these is a common cause of dyspareunia.
    D. Vaginal dryness

112. Which of the following hemoglobin A1c (HbA1c) values demonstrates control of diabetes mellitus type 2?
    A. < 7%
    B. < 8%
    C. < 6%
    D. < 9%

113. Which of the following exams can be completed by the primary care nurse practitioner during an office visit to evaluate for Alzheimer's disease?
    A. Romberg's test
    B. Rinne test
    C. Clock test
    D. Mini–mental state exam (MMSE)

114. A 65-year-old male is placed on an ACE inhibitor for hypertension control. Which of the following laboratory values should be monitored?
    A. Potassium and creatinine
    B. Potassium and sodium
    C. Potassium and magnesium
    D. Cortisol and potassium

115. Which of the following is a risk factor for *Clostridium difficile* infection?

    A. Poor hand hygiene

    B. Recent antibiotic usage

    C. Chronic constipation

    D. Consumption of contaminated water

116. Which of the following diagnoses must be reported to local health departments?

    A. Recurrent streptococcal infection

    B. Syphilis

    C. Hypertension

    D. Past Lyme disease

117. A 30-year-old female presents with complaints of linear pain around her right scapula for 5 days. She states that a burning, pustule-like rash appeared at the site 2 days ago. She has a history of chickenpox as a child. Which of the following is a likely diagnosis?

    A. Seborrheic dermatitis

    B. Impetigo

    C. Bullous dermatitis

    D. Herpes zoster

118. A 45-year-old male with a history of alcohol abuse presents with severe epigastric pain, jaundiced skin color, nausea, and vomiting. The patient is most likely suffering from which of the following conditions?

    A. Ulcer disease

    B. Cholecystitis

    C. Gastroenteritis

    D. Pancreatitis

119. Which of the following laboratory results would *not* be expected in the patient described in question 118?

    A. Decreased amylase and lipase

    B. Leukocytosis

    C. Elevated liver function panel

    D. Elevated amylase and lipase

120. Which of the following is *not* true of antibody values?

    A. IgG demonstrates past infection.

    B. IgE demonstrates allergic inflammation.

    C. IgE demonstrates severe infection.

    D. IgM demonstrates current infection.

121. Which of the following is a common treatment for osteopenia?

    A. Vitamin D with calcium and weight-bearing exercises

    B. Alendronate

    C. Vitamin D and weight-bearing exercises

    D. Calcium and alendronic acid

122. A 70-year-old retired farmer presents with a shiny gray lesion on his upper lip. The lesion measures approximately 0.5 cm × 1.0 cm × 0.3 cm. The patient states that the lesion occasionally bleeds when rubbed. Which of the following is a likely diagnosis?

    A. Squamous cell carcinoma

    B. Basal cell carcinoma

    C. Seborrheic dermatitis

    D. Malignant melanoma

123. Which of the following is the best course of treatment for the patient described in question 122?

    A. Referral to a dermatologist

    B. Topical steroid

    C. Oral antibiotic

    D. Topical antifungal

124. A 25-year-old male presents with a severe rash on his face and is diagnosed with erysipelas. Which of the following is the most common bacterial cause of this condition?

    A. *Streptococcus pyogenes*

    B. *Staphylococcus aureus*

    C. *Streptococcus agalactiae*

    D. *Escherichia coli*

125. Which of the following are the two clinical exams for meningitis that can be performed by the primary care nurse practitioner in the clinical setting?

    A. Kernig's sign and Brudzinski's sign

    B. Rovsing's sign and Kernig's sign

    C. Rinne test and Kernig's sign

    D. Brudzinski's sign and Rovsing's sign

126. Which of the following is the most common cause of death from cancer in women in the United States?

    A. Colon cancer

    B. Lung cancer

    C. Breast cancer

    D. Cervical cancer

127. A 30-year-old female presents with complaints of thin, gray vaginal discharge and pelvic pressure and is diagnosed with trichomoniasis. Which of the following is an appropriate treatment?

    A. Metronidazole

    B. Trimethoprim/sulfamethoxazole

    C. Oral antifungal

    D. Topical clindamycin

128. The patient described in question 127 reports drinking 3-4 glasses of wine every day. Which of the following is the most appropriate course of action with regard to her trichomoniasis treatment?

    A. No treatment modification is required.

    B. Initiate probiotics.

    C. Discontinue metronidazole.

    D. Recommend Alcoholics Anonymous

129. Which of the following foods should be avoided in patients taking warfarin for deep vein thrombosis?

    A. Stir-fried beef

    B. Penne and chicken

    C. Pizza

    D. Salad

130. Which of the following pieces of legislation is responsible for allowing nurse practitioners to practice in their given states?

    A. Board of nursing protocols

    B. State nurse powers acts

    C. Hospital-based protocols

    D. American Nurses Association guidelines

131. Which cranial nerves are responsible for the movement and sensation of the facial muscles?

    A. V and VII

    B. II, IV, and VI

    C. I and II

    D. X, XI, XII

132. A 40-year-old female presents with unilateral headache and lacrimation for 2-3 days. She has experienced several headaches of short duration. Which of the following types of headache is the most likely diagnosis?

    A. Cluster headache

    B. Tension headache

    C. Migraine headache

    D. Sinus headache

133. Which of the following is the best treatment for a patient with a cluster-type headache?

    A. Narcotic analgesic

    B. Oxygen therapy

    C. Tricyclic antidepressant

    D. Triptan therapy

134. A nurse working at a local emergency department presents for a PPD test. She returns 2 days later for her results with an 11 mm erythema and induration. What is this reading considered?

    A. Negative

    B. Positive

    C. The test requires a second step.

    D. Indeterminate

135. A 27-year-old female presents for dizziness with position changes. Her vital signs are stable, and the physical exam is benign except for sinus congestion on visual exam of the nares. She states that she had a viral upper respiratory infection one week ago. Which of the following is the most likely diagnosis?

    A. Benign positional vertigo

    B. Dizziness of unknown origin

    C. Dizziness with a neurological cause

    D. Ménière's disease

136. Why is a mammogram occasionally inconclusive in younger female patients?
    A. Poor quality of mammogram
    B. Dense breast tissue
    C. Irregular menstrual cycles
    D. Irregularities in breast tissue

137. Which type of consent is given in emergency situations when no one is present to give consent on the patient's behalf when the patient has no decision making capacity?
    A. Informed consent
    B. Implied consent
    C. Life-or-death consent
    D. Emergency consent

138. Which of the following is *not* a potential cause of seizure?
    A. Hyponatremia or hypernatremia
    B. Hypoxia
    C. Hyperglycemia
    D. Alcohol withdrawal

139. A 30-year-old nonsmoker presents for persistent dyspnea. There are no overt signs of asthma or other reversible conditions. A diagnosis of COPD, emphysema type, is made. Which of the following is the most likely cause?
    A. Second-hand smoke
    B. Environmental causes
    C. Alpha-1 antitrypsin deficiency
    D. Vitamin deficiency

140. Which of the following is *not* an autoimmune disease?
    A. Rheumatoid arthritis
    B. Osteoarthritis
    C. Hashimoto's thyroiditis
    D. Systemic lupus erythematosus

141. Which of the following medications is the best treatment for chronic gout management in a person with renal insufficiency?
    A. Ibuprofen
    B. Colchicine
    C. Febuxostat
    D. Allopurinol

142. Which of the following is *not* a sign of active tuberculosis?
    A. Fever
    B. Cough
    C. Weight gain
    D. Night sweats

143. A patient from the Dominican Republic tests positive for tuberculosis via skin test. Following a positive interferon gamma release assay (IGRA) serum assay and negative chest X-ray, which of the following is the most appropriate next step?
    A. Infectious disease consultation
    B. Vancomycin
    C. No treatment is required.
    D. Isoniazid and vitamin B6

144. A 27-year-old male presents with wheezing and a reddened face. He states he has just been stung by a bee but that he has never had an allergy before. Which of the following is the most likely diagnosis?
    A. Asthma exacerbation
    B. Anaphylaxis
    C. Allergic reaction to bee sting
    D. Facial cellulitis

145. Which of the following is an appropriate medication for the patient described in question 144?
    A. Epinephrine via auto-injector
    B. Intramuscular methylprednisolone sodium succinate
    C. Oral diphenhydramine
    D. Intramuscular diphenhydramine

146. Which of the following is the document that outlines a patient's wishes in the event that they are no longer able to speak for themselves?
    A. Advanced directive or living will
    B. Do-not-resuscitate (DNR) order
    C. Power of attorney
    D. Do-not-intubate (DNI) order

147. Nurse practitioners are allowed to bill for their services at which of the following?
    A. 100% under their own national provider identity number
    B. 85% under their own national provider identity number
    C. 85% under their collaborating physician's national provider identity number
    D. Nurse practitioners are not able to bill for their services.

148. Who was responsible for the first nurse practitioner program?
    A. Loretta Ford
    B. Sister Callista Roy
    C. Clara Barton
    D. Florence Nightingale

149. Which of the following foods is considered safe for a patient taking a monoamine oxidase inhibitor (MAOI)?
    A. Red wine
    B. Cured meat
    C. Dark, leafy vegetables
    D. Hard cheese

150. A 29-year-old female presents reporting that she has missed 2 days of her oral birth control medication and is concerned that she will not be protected. What is the best advice for this patient?
    A. Restart the medication immediately, but also use another form of birth control.
    B. Stop taking the medication for this month, and resume next month.
    C. Continue the medication; no other intervention required.
    D. Another form of birth control should be used entirely.

Adult Test Answers

INTRODUCTION

1. A. Trimethoprim/sulfamethoxazole

   The only medication of the options given that is contraindicated in a history of G6PD deficiency is trimethoprim/sulfamethoxazole. All other medications are safe. Sulfa drugs act as an oxidant stress on the red cell membrane. In an individual without G6PD deficiency, there is enough glutathione reductase to counteract this oxidant stress. In G6PD deficiency, red cells are destroyed. The most common oxidant stress leading to hemolysis in G6PD deficiency is infection.

2. A. Urinalysis

   This patient appears to be demonstrating signs and symptoms of a urinary tract infection, which is most likely pyelonephritis because of the flank pain. A urinalysis is the most appropriate exam to determine if this diagnosis is correct. The presence of white cells on urinalysis is more specific than bacteria in determining the presence of a urinary tract infection.

3. D. Fifth intercostal space, left midclavicular line

   The second intercostal space on the right sternal border is the aortic valve; the third intercostal space is Erb's point. Murmurs of mitral regurgitation are best heard at the apex, where the nipple is located on the left side of the chest. Murmurs of mitral regurgitation radiate to the axilla.

4. A. Metformin

   Metformin is recognized as the first-line medication for type 2 diabetes mellitus, unless the patient is intolerant to the medication. Patients with type 2 diabetes are often not initiated on insulin until treatment with all oral medications is exhausted. Metformin works by inhibiting gluconeogenesis. This is why metformin does not cause hypoglycemia. Metformin does not cause weight gain. Sulfonylureas and rosiglitazone both cause weight gain. The most common contraindication to metformin is renal insufficiency. Metformin occasionally causes lactic acidosis in those with renal insufficiency.

5. B. Hypothyroidism

   Hypothyroidism is characterized by feeling cold; dry, brittle hair; and weight gain. Thyroid hormone is the main reason body temperature is maintained at a constant 36.7°C even in cold environments. Patients with hyperthyroidism usually feel warm. Patients with hypertension and hyperglycemia do not usually report the complaints of the patient in this question.

6. D. TSH up and T4 down

When a patient has hypothyroidism, TSH is elevated. The higher the number for TSH is up, the more the size of the gland is down. Almost all hypothyroidism is caused by a gland that has become underactive as a result of the inflammation of Hashimoto's thyroiditis. When the gland is underactive, T4 (thyroxine) production goes down. When T4 production goes down, the pituitary gland increases its secretion of TSH.

7. B. Penicillin

Penicillin is still recognized as the primary first-line treatment for streptococcal pharyngitis. Amoxicillin and penicillin V potassium (penicillin VK) are just as good as any other medication. If the patient is penicillin allergic, other medications are used. If the allergy is a rash, cephalexin is used. If the allergy is anaphylaxis, azithromycin is used. Cephalosporins are safe to use if the penicillin allergy results only in a rash.

8. A. Rash is a known side effect of penicillin when used in mononucleosis.

There is about a 30-40% incidence of rash among those treated with penicillin-based antibiotics for mononucleosis. This is not an idiopathic infection. The rash could be an allergic reaction, but the question clearly states there are no signs or symptoms of allergic reaction. A rash can signal a potential life-threatening emergency, but, again, no indication of such is given in the question.

9. C. Amlodipine

Amlodipine is a calcium channel blocker indicated for isolated systolic hypertension. The other options may all work, but amlodipine is the best option. Beta blockers are the first line of therapy in hypertension only in patients with coronary artery disease or congestive heart failure.

10. A. A collaborative agreement requires electronic supervision at all times.

In most states that require a collaborative agreement, the agreement stipulates that the collaborative physician (or his or her designee) must maintain electronic communication at all times. A collaborative agreement does not require direct supervision. Supervisory agreements require direct supervision.

11. B. Liver function tests (LFTs)

Prior to initiating oral antifungal therapy, a complete metabolic profile including LFTs should be completed and then monitored throughout therapy.

12. D. Angiotensin-converting enzyme (ACE) inhibitor or angiotensin receptor blocker (ARB)

An ACE inhibitor or ARB is indicated as the primary medication for hypertensive therapy in diabetes management as these medications offer renal protection. An ACE inhibitor is also indicated as first-line therapy in patients with hypertension and proteinuria. Diabetes alone, without hypertension or proteinuria, is not an indication for an ACE inhibitor.

13. C. Oseltamivir

Oseltamivir is the only medication indicated for the treatment of influenza. Azithromycin and penicillin are indicated for bacterial infections. Neuraminidase inhibitors such oseltamivir are useful in the first 48 hours after the onset of symptoms.

14. A. Statin and acetylsalicylic acid (Aspirin)

All patients discharged from the hospital should be initiated on a statin and acetylsalicylic acid unless there is a contraindication or other medications are prescribed in their stead. If the patient is already on aspirin either add dipyridamole or switch the acetylsalicylic acid to clopidogrel. Both recommendations are for cases of nonhemorrhagic stroke.

15. A. Parkinson's disease

Resting tremor, bradykinesia, rigidity, and gait instability present the clear picture of Parkinson's disease. Cerebral vascular accident and transient ischemic attack are more acute processes, and neither produces tremor and rigidity.

16. B. Myelin sheath

Multiple sclerosis is the destruction of the myelin sheath, the protective coating of the neurons. This causes progressively worsening and decreased motor functioning. Lewy bodies are present in Lewy body dementia and in certain cases of Alzheimer's disease.

17. C. Pyelonephritis

Flank pain with fever and dysuria are indicative of pyelonephritis. A lower urinary tract infection does not usually produce flank pain or fever. Neither gastroenteritis nor colitis fit this clinical picture. Diagnosis is confirmed with a urinalysis showing white blood cells and a CT scan showing enlargement of the kidneys.

18. B. Levofloxacin

Levofloxacin is a common outpatient therapy for pyelonephritis as it covers both the upper and lower urinary tract. The other medications listed cover pathogens specific to the lower urinary tract. Cephalexin, nitrofurantoin, and trimethoprim/sulfamethoxazole (TMP/SMX) are all good choices for cystitis, but are not as beneficial for pyelonephritis.

19. A. Rhabdomyolysis

Rhabdomyolysis is the breakdown of muscle tissue, which is characterized by tea-colored urine and red blood cells in the urine. The use of protein shakes and extreme exercise can exacerbate this condition. Myoglobin, hemoglobin, and red blood cells will all be positive on urine dipstick. Only on microscopic examination can it be proved that it is myoglobin causing the dipstick to be positive for blood.

20. C. Acetylcholine

Myasthenia gravis is a neurological condition affecting acetylcholine. Receptors for acetylcholine are lost exclusively at the neuromuscular junction. There is absolutely no effect in the brain with myasthenia gravis. The best initial test is an acetylcholine receptor antibody test. The best initial therapy is either pyridostigmine or neostigmine, both of which inhibit acetylcholine esterase and increase acetylcholine levels at the neuromuscular junction.

21. A. The dose should be increased.

If TSH is elevated, the gland is underactive (hypothyroidism), and the patient requires greater hormone supplementation. Measuring TSH and T4 levels are the two ways of assessing whether the dosage of thyroid hormone replacement is sufficient. The dose of levothyroxine (synthetic thyroid hormone replacement) should be increased until the patient's TSH levels are normal. Dosage is usually adjusted at intervals of every 3 to 6 weeks.

22. C. 150/90 mm Hg

A reading of 150/90 mm Hg or above is considered by the JNC 8 guidelines to indicate the need for blood pressure control in patients over 60 years of age. For those under age 60, with or without diabetes, the goal for blood pressure is 140/90 mm Hg.

23. B. Hydrochlorothiazide

Thiazide diuretics are common antihypertensives. Carvedilol, diltiazem, or labetalol may be used as a first-line therapy in certain situations.

24. A. Second intercostal space, right side; systolic murmur

This is the location of the aortic valve. An aortic stenosis murmur is a systolic murmur. This murmur will radiate to the carotid arteries. The murmur of pulmonic stenosis is heard at the second left intercostal space. The murmur of aortic regurgitation is heard at the lower left sternal border.

25. A. Acute gastroenteritis

This question describes the clinical picture of acute gastroenteritis. Blood in the stool may signify a bacterial origin, but that is not what the question is asking about. Crohn's disease and irritable bowel syndrome do not present acutely. Cholecystitis never presents with blood in the stool. Cholecystitis presents with right upper quadrant abdominal pain with tenderness to palpation. Irritable bowel syndrome never presents with blood in the stool. Irritable bowel syndrome rarely presents with vomiting. It is possible that this could be a first episode of Crohn's disease or ulcerative colitis, but infectious gastroenteritis is much more common.

26. C. Stool cultures

Prior to starting antibiotics, stool cultures should be obtained so that the appropriate etiology of the infection can be identified and, if indicated, the appropriate antibiotic can be selected. *Always remember: assessment before treatment.* This does not mean you have to wait for the results of the culture to initiate treatment, but you must obtain the culture. Further, you should not initiate an antispasmodic agent, such as diphenoxylate, until antibiotics have been given.

27. D. Left lower quadrant

The most common site of pain associated with diverticulitis is the left lower quadrant. Right lower quadrant pain is associated with appendicitis, right upper quadrant pain with cholecystitis, and left upper quadrant pain with gastritis. An elevated white cell count and fever in addition to pain suggest diverticulitis. A CT scan is the confirmatory test for diverticulitis. A colonoscopy should *not* be performed for diverticulitis, as there is an increased risk of perforation in diverticulitis compared to those with only diverticulosis.

28. C. Referral for colonoscopy

Colonoscopy is part of routine management for a 50-year-old male. Neither a PSA test nor a DRE is routine any longer; there is simply no good screening test for prostate cancer. One-quarter of those with an elevated PSA level do not have prostate cancer, and one-quarter of those with prostate cancer do not have an elevated PSA level. The use of PSA testing and DRE does not lower prostate cancer mortality. The herpes zoster (shingles) vaccine is not indicated until age 60.

29. D. Muscle cramps

Muscle cramps are a common complaint associated with hypokalemia. Tachycardia, bloody stool, and dysuria are not associated with hypokalemia. Low potassium levels interfere with the depolarization of myocytes.

30. D. Ketones

Ketones are seen when fat is broken down by the body instead of glucose; this is commonly seen in dehydration and uncontrolled diabetes. Bacteria, leukocytes, and nitrites are all associated with urinary tract infections. The most important of these findings is leucocytes. If there is fever, dysuria, and pain, then the presence of white cells alone is sufficient to diagnose a urinary tract infection.

31. D. Between −1.0 and −2.5

    A T score between −1.0 and −2.5 is considered osteopenia. A score of −2.5 or less is considered osteoporosis. The other options given are not associated with either of those conditions. Bone densitometry is routinely recommended for all women beginning at age 65.

32. A. Viral upper respiratory infection

    According to the description provided in the question, the patient most likely has a viral syndrome. There is nothing in the question to indicate sinusitis, pneumonia, or streptococcal pharyngitis.

33. A. Combination decongestant/expectorant

    As this condition is suspected to be viral, antibiotics are not indicated; supportive therapy is the best course of treatment.

34. A. Azithromycin

    First-line therapy for community-acquired pneumonia (CAP) is azithromycin. Penicillin and amoxicillin are not indicated for CAP. Vancomycin is usually reserved for severe nosocomial infection.

35. A. About halfway between the right iliac crest and the umbilicus

    McBurney's point, associated with the location of the appendix, is located about halfway between the right iliac crest and the umbilicus. The right upper quadrant is associated with the gall bladder or liver. The left lower quadrant is associated with diverticulitis. Right lower quadrant pain near the pubic bone might indicate an ovarian cyst.

36. B. Phalen's test

    Phalen's test evaluates for carpel tunnel syndrome. The test is conducted by the patient pressing the hands against each other in extreme flexion to put pressure on the carpal tunnel. The Finklestein test evaluates for De Quervain tenosynovitis. The anterior drawer test evaluates for knee instability. McBurney's point tenderness indicates appendicitis.

37. B. Ibuprofen

    NSAIDs such as ibuprofen are used as first-line pain relief therapy for joint complaints from inflammation such as the epicondylitis of exercise or tennis elbow. Oxycodone is used for refractory pain. Nonpharmacologic therapies are used in conjuncture with pharmacologic therapies. Acetaminophen may be used in NSAID-allergic or NSAID-intolerant patients. Acetaminophen is used for the pain of osteoarthritis. In osteoarthritis, the pain does not result from inflammation. In addition, since osteoarthritis requires daily pain medication, there is a real risk of ulcer disease with the daily use of NSAIDs.

38. A. Hydrocele

    A hydrocele is a fluid-filled cyst in the scrotum visible under transillumination. A spermatocele is a collection of fluid containing immature sperm cells. A varicocele is an enlargement of the pampiniform venous plexus. No treatment is needed for a hydrocele.

39. D. Testicular torsion

    Testicular torsion is an emergent condition that must be addressed within 6 hours of onset. Testicular cancer and epididymitis typically do not present acutely. Urinary tract infections do not present with testicular pain. Testicular torsion presents with an elevated testicle because the twisting shortens the spermatic cord. The only treatment is to surgically unwind the spermatic cord.

40. A. Immediate emergency department referral

This patient has approximately 6 hours from the onset of testicular torsion to undergo surgery before the testicle is likely die. No other option given addresses the emergent nature of this condition.

41. B. Cauda equina syndrome

Cauda equina syndrome is a medical emergency in which the lumbar plexus ceases to function. Bowel and bladder incontinence is common, and saddle (hence "equina") anesthesia (buttock numbness) is a staple of the condition. Cauda equina syndrome can also be caused by metastatic cancer.

42. C. Neuroleptic malignant syndrome

The presenting symptoms in conjunction with the medications the patient is taking (risperidone and tramadol) are very concerning for neuroleptic malignant syndrome (NMS). This condition should be considered an emergency. NMS and malignant hyperthermia are both considered idiosyncratic reactions to medications. NMS occurs as a result of antipsychotic medications; malignant hyperthermia occurs as a result of anesthetics. Both present with fever, muscle destruction, and an increased CPK level. Both NMS and malignant hyperthermia are treated with dantrolene. NMS is also treated with dopamine agonists such as bromocriptine or cabergoline.

43. A. Bipolar disorder

Bipolar disorder is a psychiatric disorder characterized by period of mania alternating with periods of depression. Bipolar 1 is characterized by the experience of at least one full manic episode. Bipolar 2 is characterized by the experience of at least one major depressive episode and one hypomanic episode but no full manic episode. Bipolar disorder is the mental illness most associated with suicide.

44. A. Untreated chlamydia

Untreated chlamydia is the leading cause of pelvic inflammatory disease. The answer would be the same if the question asked about urethritis or cervicitis.

45. A. Azithromycin

Azithromycin is recommended by the Centers for Disease Control and Prevention (CDC) as the primary treatment for uncomplicated chlamydia infection (provided the patient is not allergic to the medication). Ceftriaxone is the first-line therapy for gonorrhea. Ciprofloxacin should be avoided because of drug resistance. Penicillin is not indicated. In general, for urethritis, cervicitis, and PID, *both* chlamydia and gonorrhea are treated for; patients receive ceftriaxone and azithromycin or doxycycline for PID.

46. D. Providing support and time to adjust to new situations and surroundings

Providing support and time to adjust to new situations and surroundings is not an example of elder abuse or neglect. The other options are all examples of elder abuse or neglect.

47. D. Hordeolum internum

A hordeolum internum is a stye on the inner eyelid. A hordeolum externum occurs on the outer eyelid. Chalazion occurs when the oil gland becomes blocked, not infected. Conjunctivitis is an inflammation of the conjunctiva, the mucous membrane that covers the front of the eye and lines the inside of the eyelids.

48. B. Topical erythromycin

Internal hordeola (infected, blocked oil glands) require topical antibiotics. External hordeola usually require oral antibiotics. Chalazia can be treated without antibiotics using warm compresses and gentle massage.

49. A. Erythema migrans

    Erythema migrans is the name for this type of rash. When a patient presents with erythema migrans (a rash shaped like a bull's eye with redness on the outside and a pale center), treatment with doxycycline or amoxicillin should be initiated immediately. The erythema migrans rash is considered so characteristic of Lyme disease that confirmatory testing with serology is typically not needed. Rosacea is a chronic skin condition. Fluid-filled pustules and Koplik spots are associated with measles.

50. D. Flu-like symptoms

    Persistent flu-like symptoms are the most common complaints associated with early HIV infection. Fever may be present, but not always. Blood in the stool and hyperactivity are not associated with the initial symptoms of HIV.

51. C. When the CD4 count is less than 200

    A CD4 count less than 200 is considered stage 3 disease or AIDS. Treatment, however, is not based on staging or CD4 count. All patients with HIV or AIDS should be treated with a combination of 3 to 4 antiretroviral medications. A common regimen consists of 2 nucleoside reverse transcriptase inhibitors, such as tenofovir and emtricitabine, in combination with an integrase inhibitor or protease inhibitor.

52. B. Periorbital cellulitis

    Periorbital cellulitis is cellulitis around the eye that has the potential to cause serious harm and paralysis to the optical nerve. Systemic infectious is also possible with this condition. Periorbital cellulitis is treated with intravenous (IV) cefazolin or vancomycin. Periorbital cellulitis is largely a skin infection. Orbital cellulitis is an infection of the globe of the eye itself.

53. C. Low hemoglobin, low hematocrit, low MCH, low MCV

    A CBC showing low hemoglobin, low hematocrit, low MCH, and low MCV is typical of iron deficiency anemia. Iron deficiency is confirmed by low iron, low ferritin, and an increased total iron-binding capacity. Iron-binding capacity measures the blood's capacity to bind iron with transferrin. A high iron-binding capacity indicates that iron levels are low.

54. A. Low hemoglobin, low hematocrit, high MCH, high MCV

    B12 deficiency interferes with red blood cell production, which results in low hemoglobin, low hematocrit, high MCH, and high MCV as part of a macrocytic anemia. Macrocytic anemia is characterized by large cells and a high MCV. B12 and folate deficiency are also characterized by megaloblastic anemia, which is a hypersegmentation of neutrophils.

55. A. Inferior vena cava, right atrium, tricuspid valve, right ventricle, pulmonary artery, lungs, pulmonary vein, left artery, mitral valve, left ventricle, aorta

    Venous return to the heart is via the right atrium from the inferior and superior venae cavae. Blood fills the right ventricle passively through the tricuspid valve. Blood leaves the right ventricle to enter the pulmonary artery. The pulmonary artery is the only artery to carry deoxygenated blood, and the pulmonary vein is the only vein to carry oxygenated blood. This is because an artery is defined as a blood vessel leaving the heart, whereas a vein is a blood vessel entering the heart.

56. B. II, III, AvF

    EKG leads II, III, and AvF are the leads that correspond to inferior myocardial ischemia and infarction. These leads represent the right ventricle. Leads I, AvL, V5, and V6 represent the lateral wall of the left ventricle. The anterior wall is assessed by leads V2-V4, which reflect perfusion through the left anterior descending artery. This is the most important artery in the sense that occlusion of this vessel results in the greatest risk of death.

57. B. Calcium channel blockers

Calcium channel blockers are not one of the mainstay treatments for congestive heart failure (CHF) as they can potentially exacerbate some symptoms. The medications that most lower mortality in CHF are those that inhibit the renin–angiotensin–aldosterone system. ACE inhibitors, beta blockers, and spironolactone all inhibit aldosterone. Beta blockers slow the heart rate and allow for increased perfusion of the coronary arteries. In addition, beta blockade inhibits the release of renin from the juxtaglomerular complex. Calcium channel blockers do not slow the sinus heart rate or decrease aldosterone, which is part of the reason they do not benefit CHF.

58. C. Edema

All answer options except for edema are characteristics of emphysema. Edema is the pooling of fluids.

59. A. *Streptococcus pyogenes*

Streptococcus pyogenes is the most common cause of impetigo. *Staphylococcus aureus* is the second most common. The *Streptococcus* strain involved in skin infections is also called group A beta-hemolytic streptococcus. Skin infections can cause glomerulonephritis, but the *Streptococcus pyogenes* isolates that affect the skin cannot cause rheumatic fever.

60. C. Ampicillin

Ampicillin given with mononucleosis may cause a rash in the patient. This rash is not life threatening but is often pruritic and can be irritating.

61. B. Angiotensin-converting enzyme (ACE) inhibitor

ACE inhibitors are used as first-line antihypertensive medications in patients with diabetes (provided there are no contraindications) because of their renal protective features. ACE inhibitors decrease the rate of progression to proteinuria. In addition, in renal insufficiency, ACE inhibitors decrease the rate of worsening of creatinine.

62. A. High fiber

Seeds are not dangerous in a patient with diverticulitis. For a long time, it was thought that seeds may cause a reoccurrence of diverticulitis, but this is not true. A patient with diverticulitis should be counseled to follow a high-fiber diet. Low salt is indicated in hypertension, and low vitamin K is indicated in patients taking anticoagulants.

63. D. Homans' sign

Homans' sign is used in the clinical evaluation of deep vein thrombosis. If this test is positive, an ultrasound is usually completed to confirm diagnosis. The problem with Homans' sign is that it lacks specificity. A lower extremity Doppler study must be performed to confirm the presence of a clot even if Homans' sign is positive.

64. B. Ankle-brachial index

The ankle-brachial index (ABI) is a clinical exam used to evaluate arterial function in suspected peripheral arterial disease. The ABI is the ratio of blood pressure at the ankle to the blood pressure in the upper arm. With the patient lying flat, the blood pressure at the ankle should be the same as the blood pressure in the upper arm; that is, the ABI should be 1.0 (equal). An ABI of less than 0.9 indicates some form of obstruction. An ABI of less than 0.5 indicates a severe obstruction.

65. C. Prophylthiouracil

Prophylthiouracil is a medication for hyperthyroidism that is considered first line in pregnant patients, especially during the first trimester. Newer studies are showing that for the second and third trimesters, patients should be transitioned to methimazole.

66. C. Vomiting

Vomiting is a common cause of hypokalemia. Gastric fluid is high in potassium, and vomiting therefore results in potassium loss. Vomiting also causes alkalosis, which drives potassium into cells and worsens the alkalosis. Renal failure results in high potassium levels because the potassium cannot be excreted. Spironolactone and ACE inhibitors increase potassium levels because they inhibit aldosterone. Aldosterone increases potassium excretion. Crush injury increases plasma potassium levels because it causes the release of intracellular potassium. Of all potassium in the body, 95% is intracellular. Anything that breaks down cells rapidly increases plasma potassium levels.

67. D. Diabetic ketoacidosis

Acute renal failure results in elevated serum potassium levels. Diabetic ketoacidosis causes high potassium for two reasons. First, insulin, which normally drives potassium intracellularly, is not present. Second, most cases of acidosis lead to potassium release from cells, particularly red blood cells. Licorice acts like aldosterone, and anything that increases aldosterone increases potassium loss from the body. Diuretics such as thiazides and furosemide block potassium absorption in the tubule.

68. D. Trichomoniasis

Trichomoniasis presents with thin, gray vaginal discharge. Yeast infection traditionally presents with thick, white, cottage cheese–like discharge. Chlamydia and gonorrhea present with green discharge or no discharge at all. Trichomoniasis and bacterial vaginitis are the two most likely conditions to cause vaginal itching. Both trichomoniasis and bacterial vaginitis are treated with metronidazole.

69. C. Yeast infection

Yeast infection typically presents with thick, white, cottage cheese–like discharge. Chlamydia and gonorrhea present with green discharge or no discharge at all. Trichomoniasis presents with thin, gray vaginal discharge. Fungal vaginitis is treated with a topical antifungal such as miconazole, clotrimazole, terconazole, or econazole. Oral fluconazole is also highly effective.

70. C. Supportive care

Hepatitis A is a self-limiting viral illness usually characterized by nausea, vomiting, and diarrhea. No oral or IV medication is required to treat the infection. However, IV medications and fluids may be required if the nausea or vomiting becomes severe. The only form of acute hepatitis that is treated is acute hepatitis C.

71. A. CAGE

CAGE stands for the following questions:

Have you ever felt you needed to **C**ut down on your drinking or drug use?

Have people **A**nnoyed you by criticizing your drinking or drug use?

Have you felt bad or **G**uilty about your drinking or drug use?

Have you ever had a drink or used drugs first thing in the morning to steady your nerves or to get rid of a hangover (**E**ye-opener)?

If the patient answers yes to one or more question, he or she should be referred to the appropriate resource.

72. A. Irritable bowel syndrome

Irritable bowel syndrome (IBS) is a psychosomatic condition in which anxiety causes physical symptoms that can mimic ulcerative colitis or Crohn's disease without blood or mucous in the stool. IBS is the most common reason for a long-term relationship with a gastroenterologist. IBS is treated initially with fiber and stool-bulking agents.

73. C. BRCA1 and BRCA2

BRCA1 and BRCA2 gene mutations are the most common genetic abnormality seen in breast cancer. Li-Fraumeni syndrome and Cowden syndrome are also associated with a higher risk of breast cancer but are less commonly involved than BRCA1 and BRCA2 gene mutations.

74. A. Cremasteric reflex

The cremasteric reflex is demonstrated when the inner thigh is stimulated, causing a retraction of the scrotum on the side stimulated. An absence of the cremasteric reflex is considered diagnostic of testicular torsion. The blue dot sign may also be seen in testicular torsion but is much less diagnostic than the absence of the cremasteric reflex.

75. C. 6 hours

A patient with ovarian torsion has about 6 hours for the ovarian torsion to be properly diagnosed and detorsed (usually surgically) to prevent loss of the ovary.

76. B. Demyelination of the neurons

Demyelination of the neurons is the cause of all types of multiple sclerosis. It is initially treated with a bolus doses of steroids if there is an acute decompensation. Long-term therapy to prevent a relapse is with beta interferon, mitoxantrone, dalfampridine, or fingolimod. It is not clear that any of the preventive agents is superior to the others. The presence of Lewy bodies is characteristic of Lewy body dementia and certain cases of Alzheimer's disease. An inflammation of the meninges is present in meningitis.

77. D. Resting tremor

A resting tremor is characteristic of Parkinson's disease. A resting tremor presents when the patient is immobile; it goes away when the patient moves. Tremor and gait disorder are the two most common symptoms of Parkinson's disease. There is no specific diagnostic test for Parkinson's disease.

78. C. VII

Cranial nerve VII, the facial nerve, is the nerve affected in Bell's palsy. Treatment is with prednisone. Hyperacute hearing and taste disturbance may also present in Bell's palsy because the seventh cranial nerve has an impact on both hearing and taste.

79. B. *Candida*

Candida is the fungus most commonly involved in intertrigo infection. In obese patients with uncontrolled diabetes, this type of infection is common in folds of fatty tissue with skin-to-skin contact.

80. D. Topical antifungal

Topical antifungals are first-line therapy for intertrigo. If topical antifungal therapy fails, an oral antifungal may be used if the situation warrants. There is no indication to use topical or oral antibiotics for a supposed fungal infection. Fungal intertrigo is treated with the same topical antifungals used to treat fungal vaginitis.

81. C. Liver function tests (LFTs)

Prior to starting terbinafine, liver function must be known. Liver function panels must also be taken during therapy.

82. D. Both conditions have allergic triggers.

Both eczema and asthma have allergic triggers and may be exacerbated by the same trigger. There is no bacterial cause for either of these conditions. If a bacterial source is suspected, asthma and eczema should not be the diagnosis.

83. D. Seborrheic dermatitis

Seborrheic dermatitis is a benign skin growth that occurs in sun-exposed locations in elderly individuals. Seborrheic dermatitis is treated with topical antifungals and sometimes topical steroids. Basal cell and squamous cell carcinomas tend to be fast growing, ulcerative, and shiny or scaly in nature.

84. A. Central vision

Macular degeneration is associated with the loss of central vision. Eventually total blindness occurs, but this is a late finding. Macular degeneration can be treated with intraocular injections of vascular endothelial growth factor (VEGF) inhibitors. Ophthalmologic referral is critical.

85. B. Refer to the emergency department

Acute angle-closure glaucoma is a medical emergency. Without emergency intervention, severe vision deterioration or loss can occur. Pilocarpine drops and beta blocker drops are required to constrict the pupil and open the canal of Schlemm. IV mannitol is also sometimes used.

86. D. Yoga

Yoga may help individuals feel better, but it is not directly therapeutic for any particular disease.

87. D. Talking

Talking cannot cause temporomandibular joint (TMJ) disorder. All other options are common causes of TMJ.

88. D. Isoniazid

Isoniazid is a common treatment for tuberculosis; it is not used in the evaluation of tuberculosis.

89. A. Asthma is reversible.

Asthma and chronic obstructive pulmonary disease (COPD) have similar obstructive properties in the lungs and yield similar complaints in patients. The treatment of each is also similar, as oral and inhaled steroids and short and long-acting beta agonists alleviate both conditions. Asthma, however, is reversible, whereas COPD is not. If it is unclear whether there is a reversible component to a patient's lung disease, pulmonary function tests (PFTs) are ordered. With a PFT, the forced expiratory volume during the first second of the forced breath (FEV1) can be measured before and after the use of an albuterol inhaler. If there is an improvement in FEV1 by at least 20%, a reversible asthmatic airway obstruction component is present.

90. D. Severe persistent asthma requires intubation.

Severe persistent asthma may require intubation but not always. All other answer choices are true of asthma.

91. D. Below 80% is abnormal.

An FEV1 value below 80% is considered abnormal. The lower the value, the greater is the obstruction. The cutoff value of 80% is also applied to the other

PFT parameters: forced vital capacity (FVC), total lung capacity (TLC), and residual volume (RV).

92. A. Obstruction

An FEV1 below 80% indicates obstruction. A poorly performed test brings the results of the evaluation into question, but there is no indication of this in the question.

93. B. The patient actively wants to quit smoking.

When the patient actively wants to quit smoking, it is the optimal time for the provider to assist the patient in smoking cessation, as this is when the patient will be most likely to succeed. Insurance coverage, family wishes, and comorbidities may also help the patient be successful, but the patient's desire to quit needs to be the driving force.

94. B. Vivid dreams

Vivid dreams are a commonly reported side effect of varenicline. It was previously thought that there was an increased risk of suicidality with varenicline, but this has proved untrue.

95. A. Call 911

A pulsatile mass may indicate an abdominal aortic aneurysm. This is an emergent condition that can be life threatening. In this case, the patient not only has a pulsatile mass but also pain.

96. C. Elevated BMI, elevated SBP, elevated triglycerides, elevated glucose, decreased HDL

These results correctly define metabolic syndrome.

97. C. 6

There are 6 grades of cardiac murmur. An I/VI murmur is heard only with auscultatory maneuvers.

98. B. 2-3

Murmurs can usually a murmur can be heard around grade 2-3. A grade 4 murmur has a palpable vibration that can be felt by touching the chest.
A palpable murmur is called a thrill.

99. A. Late-systolic click

Late-systolic click is the correct description of a murmur associated with mitral valve prolapse. The click is followed by the murmur of mitral regurgitation. Early-diastolic blowing is associated with pulmonary regurgitation. A late-diastolic click is associated with complete heart block.

100. C. Admission to hospital for observation

Observation admissions are short-term, and of the 4 options, this provides the least amount of risk for deep vein thrombosis.

101. A. Dark stool

Dark, almost black, stool can be noted with pink bismuth. This black stool can be distinguished from bloody stool with the fecal occult blood test. Bismuth is heme negative. Red stool, fever, and right lower quadrant pain are all associated with potentially emergent situations.

102. A. Strict blood pressure control

Strict blood pressure control, usually with alpha and beta blockade, is required prior to the removal of a pheochromocytona. This is because of the additional stress hormones secreted by this tumor. The agent most often used is the alpha blocker phenoxybenzamine, given intravenously.

103. D. To decrease the adherence of bacteria to tissue

Cranberry juice acts as a tissue barrier and blocks bacteria from adhering to the tissue of the lower urinary tract. However, it is unclear whether this is truly effective in a clinical infection.

104. C. Diuretics

Diuretics are not a cause of erectile dysfunction. Stress, benign prostatic hyperplasia, and diabetes, especially if uncontrolled, can all cause erectile dysfunction.

105. B. Prostatitis

This clinical picture clearly defines prostatitis. Urinary tract infections do not usually present with fever or rectal pain. There is no flank pain, which is commonly seen in pyelonephritis. There is no abdominal pain, nausea, vomiting, or diarrhea as commonly seen with colitis. Prostatitis is confirmed by a tender prostate on rectal examination.

106. C. *Streptococcus pneumoniae*

Streptococcus pneumoniae is a common bacterium found in the upper respiratory tract and lungs, not in the urinary or gastrointestinal tract. The organisms that cause prostatitis are very similar to those that cause cystitis and pyelonephritis.

107. A. Lung cancer

Lung cancer is the second most common cancer among both men and women in the United States. Skin cancer is the most common. Lung cancer is the most common cause of death from cancer, but it is not the most commonly occurring cancer.

108. A. 3.5-5.0 mEq/L

While variations exist (eg, 3.5-5.5 mEq/L), this is the most commonly used reference range for potassium.

109. B. 135-145 mEq/L

135-145 mEq/L is the normal range for sodium in the body.

110. B. Ibuprofen

An NSAID such as ibuprofen is the best first-line medication for acute gouty inflammation. If NSAIDs cannot be tolerated because of ulcer disease or renal insufficiency, the next best treatment for an acute gout attack is a glucocorticoid. Colchicine is used only if NSAIDs or steroids cannot be used. Allopurinol and febuxostat are used for chronic gout management to prevent flare-ups.

111. B. Urinary tract infection

Urinary tract infections are not a common cause of dyspareunia. Sexually transmitted diseases and vaginal dryness are.

112. A. < 7%

As per the American Diabetes Association guidelines, an HbA1c value of less than 7% is considered glycemic control for those with diabetes. A diagnosis of diabetes is confirmed by an HgA1c value above 6.5%, but good control is considered to be achieved with an HgA1c value of less than 7%.

113. D. Mini–mental state exam (MMSE)

The MMSE consists of a series of questions to test the cognitive ability of individuals suspected of Alzheimer's disease or other forms of dementia. This is not the only test used for diagnosis, however.

114. A. Potassium and creatinine

ACE inhibitors, such as enalapril and lisinopril, can elevate potassium and creatinine levels, so these laboratory values should be routinely monitored.

115. B. Recent antibiotic usage

Recent antibiotic usage is a common cause of *Clostridium difficile* infection. Poor hand hygiene has ramifications for all types of infection, and contaminated water is also a common source of infection. Chronic constipation is not associated with *Clostridium difficile*. Initial therapy is with metronidazole.

116. B. Syphilis

It is mandatory to report cases of syphilis and other sexually transmitted diseases to state or city health departments. Current Lyme disease infection also requires notification. Streptococcal infections and hypertension do not require notification.

117. D. Herpes zoster

Herpes zoster (shingles) presents as burning pain in a localized site, followed by a pustule-like rash that follows a dermatome. Treatment is with oral valacyclovir, famciclovir, or acyclovir. The most accurate diagnostic test for equivocal cases is a polymerase chain reaction (PCR) of the fluid from a vesicle. Tzanck preparation has a very high false-negative rate.

118. D. Pancreatitis

Pancreatitis is an inflammation of the pancreas. Pancreatitis may result from cholelithiasis or cholecystitis but may also be caused by chronic alcohol abuse. Gastroenteritis does not usually cause jaundice and produces diffuse gastrointestinal pain. Cholecystitis rarely causes jaundice. When a stone comes out of the gallbladder and obstructs the common bile duct and pancreatic duct, both obstructive jaundice and pancreatitis result.

119. A. Decreased amylase and lipase

An elevated white blood cell count, liver function tests, amylase, and lipase would be expected in the patient with pancreatitis. As a reminder, patients with chronic severe pancreatitis may have little or no enzyme elevation toward the end of their pathology as a result of a lack of enzymes and severe tissue damage.

120. C. IgE demonstrates severe infection.

IgE usually demonstrates allergic response. All other answers are true of antibody values.

121. A. Vitamin D with calcium and weight-bearing exercises

Vitamin D with calcium and weight-bearing exercises aids in osteopenia as it helps to preserve bone function and promote new growth. Osteoporosis is treated with bisphosphonates such alendronate, pamidronate, and zoledronic acid.

122. B. Basal cell carcinoma

This is the classic clinical presentation of basal cell carcinoma. Squamous cell carcinoma looks more ulcerated with a vessel or wart-like appearance.

123. A. Referral to a dermatologist

This patient likely has skin cancer. A dermatologist will extract the lesion and have it biopsied to aid in diagnosis and treatment. Hematology and oncology can be consulted as indicated.

124. A. *Streptococcus pyogenes*

    Streptococcus pyogenes, also known as group A streptococcus, is the most common cause of erysipelas. Other causes include *Staphylococcus*.

125. A. Kernig's sign and Brudzinski's sign

    These are the two clinical exams associated with meningitis. A positive Kernig's sign consists of pain on knee extension and leg and head spasms when the body is bent forward. A positive Brudzinski's sign consists of the involuntary lifting of the legs when the head is lifted.

126. B. Lung cancer

    Breast cancer is the second most common cause of cancer-related death in women in the United States. Lung cancer is the most common cause of cancer-related death in both men and women. Almost twice as many women die of lung cancer as die of breast cancer in the United States.

127. A. Metronidazole

    Of those listed, metronidazole is the most appropriate medication for the treatment of trichomoniasis. Remember that the patient's sexual partner must also be treated.

128. C. Discontinue metronidazole

    Metronidazole has a disulfiram effect, which means that is causes an adverse reaction with alcohol similar to that caused by medications used for the treatment of alcohol abuse.

129. D. Salad

    While salad is the healthiest of the options listed, it is high in vitamin K, which can reverse the effects of warfarin. Patients are advised to limit the amount of vitamin K in their diet while on warfarin. (Treatment guidelines suggest that if a patient is on a regular diet of salads, the warfarin dosage should be modified to account for the vitamin K intake.) This interaction is one of many reasons to use factor Xa inhibitors for both clots and to prevent stroke in atrial fibrillation. Rivaroxaban, apixaban, and edoxaban have better efficacy for stroke prevention, fewer adverse effects, and fewer food interactions.

130. B. State nurse powers acts

    While there is federal legislation regarding nurse practitioners, individual state nurse powers acts govern nurse practitioners in each state. Hospital protocols and board of nursing protocols factor into the practice of nurse practitioners as well.

131. A. V and VII

    Cranial nerves V and VII are responsible for movement and sensation in the facial musculature. Cranial nerves I and II are responsible for smell and vision. Cranial nerves IV and VI aid with eye movement. Cranial nerves X, XI, and XII move the tongue, head, and shoulders. Disease of the fifth cranial nerve, trigeminal neuralgia, is profoundly painful and is treated with carbamazepine.

132. A. Cluster headache

    Cluster headaches present unilaterally, usually in the temporal area, and have unilateral lacrimation.

133. D. Triptan therapy

    Triptans are the best initial therapy to abort both migraine and cluster headaches. Triptans are contraindicated in pregnancy and in those with coronary artery disease. Although 100% oxygen is also effective, it is difficult for patients to obtain 100% oxygen for home use. Narcotic medications should be used only when all other treatment options have failed.

134. B. Positive

This test is considered positive, as the induration is 11 mm. An induration of more than 10 mm is considered positive. For those who are immunocompromised, an induration of more than 5 mm is considered positive. For the general population, an induration of more than 15 mm is considered positive.

135. A. Benign positional vertigo

Benign positional vertigo is a common complaint after a viral illness. It is caused by an imbalance of fluid in the inner ear. Treatment is with meclizine. Repositioning the head to reorient the otoliths of the ear using the Dix–Hallpike maneuver is also effective.

136. B. Dense breast tissue

Dense breast tissue, usually seen in younger females, can negatively influence the quality of a mammogram. A poor quality of mammogram can happen at any age. Irregular menstrual cycles have no implication on mammography quality. Breast tissue irregularities are what is being evaluated in a mammogram.

137. B. Implied consent

Implied consent is said to be given when the patient is unable to give consent and there is no one else available to give consent, but the provider feels that the patient's actions (ie, seeking care prior to becoming unable to give consent) indicate that he or she would want care rendered.

138. C. Hyperglycemia

Hypoglycemia, not hyperglycemia, is a cause of seizure. The other options are potential causes of seizure. Seizures are caused by disorders of sodium, oxygen, calcium, and magnesium and either liver or renal failure.

139. C. Alpha-1 antitrypsin deficiency

Alpha-1 antitrypsin deficiency is a genetic abnormality that can cause emphysema in a young individual without a history of smoking.

140. B. Osteoarthritis.

Osteoarthritis is a degenerative condition, not an autoimmune condition. It occurs from long-term wear and tear on bony structures. The other options are all autoimmune conditions.

141. C. Febuxostat

Febuxostat is a new and statistically proven most-effective medication for the long-term prevention of gouty flare-ups. Unlike allopurinol, it can be used in patients with chronic kidney disease. Ibuprofen and colchicine are used in acute gouty attacks.

142. C. Weight gain

Weight loss, not weight gain, is seen with acute tuberculosis.

143. D. Isoniazid and vitamin B6

This patient has latent tuberculosis, and, as per CDC guidelines, should be treated with isoniazid and vitamin B6 for the prevention of peripheral neuropathy. An infectious disease consultation is usually recommended, but starting the patient on the proper medication is the priority.

144. B. Anaphylaxis

This is a clear picture of acute anaphylaxis; bee stings are a common cause of anaphylaxis. There is no indication in the question of asthma or cellulitis.

145. A. Epinephrine via auto-injector

An epinephrine auto-injector is the best option for this patient as it produces the most rapid relief of anaphylaxis symptoms. Intramuscular methylpredniso-lone sodium succinate and oral diphenhydramine may also be used but not as first-line medications. Epinephrine works the fastest and is more potent than an antihistamine. However, epinephrine should *not* be used in coronary artery disease, as it will precipitate vasospasm.

146. A. Advanced directive or living will

An advanced directive or living will can only be written by a person of sound mind. It is a legal, witnessed document created by the patient stating the patient's wishes for healthcare in the event he or she becomes unable to speak for him or herself.

147. B. 85% under their own national provider identity number

Based on current reimbursement guidelines, a nurse practitioner may bill for their services at 85% of the fee schedule a physician may bill for.

148. A. Loretta Ford, PhD

Loretta Ford, PhD, and Henry Silver, MD, created the first pediatric nurse practitioner program at the University of Colorado in 1965.

149. C. Dark, leafy vegetables

While not safe for those on warfarin, dark, leafy vegetables are perfectly safe for those taking an MAOI. The other medications listed can all cause hypertensive urgency as a result of the sudden increase in tyramine.

150. A. Restart the medication immediately, but also use another form of birth control.

Hormonal birth control should be resumed as soon as possible; however, a second method of birth control should also be used for the rest of the current cycle.

Index

Page numbers followed by "f" denote figures; those followed by "t" denote tables